The Human Side of Diabetes

THE HUMAN SIDE

OF DIABETES

Beyond Doctors, Diets, and Drugs

Mike Raymond

The Noble Press
Chicago

Printed in the United States of America

Library of Congress Cataloging-in-Publication Data

Raymond, Michael W.
    The human side of diabetes : beyond doctors, diets, and drugs / Mike Raymond.
       p. cm.
    Includes bibliographical references and index.
    ISBN 1-879360-09-8 : $13.95
    1. Diabetes—Psychological aspects. I. Title
RC660.R33 1992
362.1'96462—dc20   91-50644
                                                                        CIP

10 9 8 7 6 5 4 3 2

Noble Press books are available in bulk at discount prices. Single
copies are available prepaid direct from the publisher:

Marketing Director
The Noble Press, Inc.
213 W. Institute Place, Suite 508
Chicago, IL 60610

For Eric and Bryan

Contents

Preface

THIS BOOK IS, if anything else, human.

First of all, it was an accident. It did not start out to be a book. It began as a single short essay, "After the Honeymoon," that I had written out of my frustration with my diabetes. I had returned home from a stay in the hospital which had included an introduction through a patient education program to the "new opportunities" available for living with diabetes. I found that my body was not doing what medical procedure said it was supposed to do. I wrote "After the Honeymoon" in an effort to try to figure out how I was going to maintain the energy and the will essential to keep battling a chronic disease I had had since I was nine years old.

As a college English teacher, I have been telling my students for years that writing can be a process for discovery that may help them work out problems, organize their thoughts, reveal their feelings, and evaluate their options. I took my own advice: I turned on my computer and began to peck away. The writing did not give me an answer to the problem of trying to live with (or is it *against?*) diabetes, but I certainly felt better. Before I knew it, I found myself writing more and more as I tried to come to terms with a chronic disease I had been trying to ignore for nearly three decades. Writing became one way, besides playing tennis or screaming, for me to deal with the human side of diabetes. It became a valuable ally whether I was undergoing open-heart surgery or retina laser surgery, suffering with a high blood sugar or ominous anxieties about the future, or doing battle with the insurance company or my sons. In fact, as I wrote about my diabetes, I discovered a great deal about being a husband for more than 23 years, a father of two, and a teacher at a small liberal arts university.

The result is this book. It has five sections: Invitation to the Human Side, Day-to-Day, Feelings, The Health-Care Team, and All the Difference. Each selection was written so that you could read it in a single sitting. Although several are on the same subject, such as insulin reactions or food, each functions as an independent unit. You need not read them in their order of appearance. In fact, you need not even read the book through section by section. Because you may have a particular interest that dominates your initial concerns—and because the titles are frequently a little (a lot?) bizarre—the Table of Contents provides a brief sketch of each selection's focus. The Index provides a listing of the book's contents according to the traditional terms associated with diabetes. However, the main idea is for you to read *The Human Side of Diabetes* as you like. As a person who lives in the twentieth century and as a person who has diabetes, I feel more comfortable with a structure that is not rigid. I think we all have had more than our share of structures and regimens! I hope that you will feel comfortable enough with this book to pick it up or put it down at will, to read it from start to finish or to skip around, to use it to deal with a particular problem or to get a good laugh and/or cry.

A second human element to this book is that it is uneven. The selections come in a variety of forms. You will find that some can be read as narratives: many tell stories about past experiences. Some selections may not be as much fun as the stories. A few provide information; some ask difficult questions of those with diabetes or of those who treat us. Sometimes I offer answers or advice, but usually I just wonder why there are so few answers. Others read like editorials or sermons, depending on how worked up I got about how people with diabetes are treated or mistreated. Two pieces, I must confess, were lectures I presented at conferences for health-care professionals who work with people with diabetes. There is a letter from a friend who tries to straighten me out. There are interviews with an endocrinologist, a diabetes nurse specialist, a nurse who teaches about living with diabetes, and a clinical nutritionist, which reveal their personal and professional perspectives on diabetes care. Four pieces are a physician's response to what I have written. Marvin C. Mengel, M.D., was my endocrinologist as I began to try to come to terms with my diabetes, so I badgered him to begin a written dialogue with me concerning some of the issues.

But the unevenness of *The Human Side of Diabetes* rests not so much on the diversity of forms and sources. It comes from the wide range of emotions which came to the surface as I wrote. This book is, for the most part, personal. I started with an experience or a feeling I had and then moved into a wider application for others with diabetes. ("Others with diabetes" includes those who have diabetes, those who live with or know someone with diabetes, and those who treat people who have diabetes.) As I indicated, this book began as an effort to deal with frustration. Over the years I have had a wide variety of experiences connected with my diabetes and my emotional responses have been as diverse as the experiences. As a result, you may feel that this book was written by at least six Mike Raymonds. Their personalities range from that of a clown to one of a manic-depressive; the emotions range from frustration to satisfaction, from anger to glee, from despair to jubilation, from fear to confidence. Some of the selections are sentimental; others are harsh. Sometimes all I could do was laugh; at other times nothing could prevent my depression. You may read one that reflects a calm, reasoned approach to a subject like food and then read the very next one that is a vehement, irrational attack on the insensitive idiots who are always trying to help me with my diet. Sometimes you will find evidence of substantial progress in my efforts to deal with medical people and discover another selection written a year later that contradicts the earlier experience. Many selections are not emotional at all, but provide straightforward information about ways of living with the human side of diabetes.

As I said, the book is uneven. It is neither entirely upbeat nor entirely downhearted. It is never consistently the same. That's human. That's the way my life with diabetes is. If nothing else, *The Human Side of Diabetes* strives to be authentic. Living with diabetes is at best an uneven experience. There are physical and emotional victories; there are physical and emotional setbacks. This book strives to document that people with diabetes are human. We have the strengths and weaknesses, hopes and fears, dreams and nightmares that everyone else has. We have lives to live, families to raise, jobs to hold, needs to fill, and feelings to work through. Like anyone else, we want to belong, are afraid of things that go "bump" in the night, and want to be "successful." When I admitted that I was a human being and that diabetes did not define me, identify me, or diminish my humanness, I felt that I had given myself permission to live the best that I could manage. That was the first and most crucial step in my coming to terms with diabetes.

I wish I had had this permission when I started my adventures with diabetes in 1955. It sure would have helped me as a child attending more than 17 schools, as a youth trying to compete in one sport or another, or as an adult striving for success as a teacher in two universities and as a consultant for some of America's most successful corporations. The experiences, it seems to me, would have been richer if I had been able to have them as a human rather than as a "diabetic."

Perhaps that is what this book is all about. Perhaps I just want to give you "permission" to be human. Whether you have diabetes, know someone with diabetes, or treat people with diabetes, I hope that upon reading this you will feel more worthwhile as a human being and a little less like a "diabetic." Oh, lots of information about diabetes and diabetes care is included. All sorts of advice also is offered. Nevertheless, for me, the primary value of *The Human Side of Diabetes* is the revelation that there are people behind the labels used to talk about those associated with diabetes: patient, doctor, nurse, dietician, wife, son, friend, mother, co-worker, health-care team.

It is the people behind such labels who helped provide *The Human Side of Diabetes* with the crucial element of its humanness. Without them, there would not have been a book. I am very grateful to them all.

Some introduced me to what I consider to be the "new approach" to diabetes treatment. They showed me a positive attitude for wellness. They shared with me the latest strategies and technologies for treating my disease. They taught me how and why to use those strategies and technologies. Together we constantly negotiated a therapeutic alliance for fighting the physical and emotional dimensions of my particular diabetes. But, most important, they always strived to treat me as an individual.

Some introduced me to myself as a person. They insisted that I recognize that I was doing the best I could. They accepted me as I am, warts and all, and thereby showed me how to try to accept myself. I never was a "diabetic" to them. They never treated me as a "diabetic." I was a person and was treated as a person. Such treatment encouraged me to try to live as a human being first and foremost. They showed me how it might be done, but always were wise enough to leave tome a sense that I could choose what I wanted and what I was willing to do.

People—not labels—encouraged me to live a full life, to live with diabetes, and to write about my love-hate relationship with life and the disease. These people are—literally and symbolically—in *The Human Side of Diabetes*.

Welcome to *The Human Side of Diabetes*. I hope this book confirms what you already know and already have experienced: you are human first and foremost, you are entitled to all of your feelings, you are not alone as a person or as a person with diabetes, you have choices about how you wish to live. However, if you are not convinced of or have not experienced the human side of diabetes, I hope this book offers you some ways for coming to terms with yourself and with the chronic disease. I hope it encourages you at least to give the human side a try. I am convinced it will make all the difference.

Acknowledgments

I wish to acknowledge the encouragement, support, and assistance of the following people whose faith in and insistence upon the human side were responsible for the completion of this book:

my co-authors—Wayne Dickson, Maggie Duvall, Eunice Maris, Marvin Mengel, Elizabeth Pippio, Eric Raymond, and Judy Raymond;

the health-care professionals who brought me out of the closet, taught me about diabetes and myself, kicked me in the pants, and had the fortitude to read and critique the manuscript in its early stages—Beth Dama Kraas, John Olson, Sandy Pollock, and Alberta Lee Wehrle;

the members of STS who are individually the best friends a person could have and collectively the ideal support group—Bruce Bradford, Jon Davies, Vincent Gould, Gary Maris, and John Schorr;

the Stetson University community—those with and without diabetes—who let me try out my ideas on them and put up with me throughout my personal struggles with the disease and the manuscript;

and Mark Harris, a friend whose talent, humanity, and faith as an exceptional editor transformed this dream into a reality.

PART I

Invitation to the Human Side

Invitation to the Human Side

IN MANY WAYS, we are a peculiar species.

While we want to struggle for our identity or a sense of place in a variety of unique ways, we usually see two choices. The most available and the most frequently chosen path is to accept the identity that society gives to us. Usually, it is the stereotype. The role or identity might be according to sex, age, occupation, nationality, or any other seemingly identifying characteristic. Identity can come with having a particular skin color or having a certain disease. Thus, one may become a woman or a boy, middle-aged or a senior citizen, a doctor or a teacher, an Italian or a Frenchman, a Southerner or a Texan, a Black or a diabetic.

A second choice that we may make is hibernation—hiding from those who label others or the conditions which pigeonhole us. We avoid the stereotype or label. We hide. We avoid "dehumanization" by not participating in society. We refuse to move about the city; we do not do regular jobs; we avoid public places for conversation, fun, or any other human contact. We sit in isolation—mental or physical—depending only upon our own resources in what we perceive to be a hostile world.

Fortunately, some do not succumb to either dehumanizing labels or isolating hibernation. By sharing their experiences with both alternatives, they manage to suggest another way to establish individual identity without sacrificing their connections with others. They tell their own stories. By telling their stories, they assert their individuality—a particular history of a particular person. The history shows that each person telling the story is an individual—a human with specific problems, fears, emotions, needs, joys, and responses. The very telling of the story documents unique perspectives, points of view, and approaches. Each individual style helps to show that it is his or her own story and therefore life.

The stories also reveal that each shares human experiences and attributes with many others. Each needs to live—eat, sleep, and move about. Each feels the need for contact—whether intimacy or just a sense of connection with others. Each searches for some sort of explanation of daily existence as well as for the meaning of life. Each can be happy and sad, courageous and afraid, idealistic and practical, kind and cruel, honest and insincere. Each can believe in something, be disillusioned, and then believe in something else. Each recognizes his or her mortality. Each knows that he or she is part of the human species.

Thus, they demonstrate that we can be unique while still sharing the characteristics of a species. They also demonstrate that, by recognizing that each person has his or her own individual story, a person can be an individual without sacrificing an identification with the human race. The personal history resolves the dilemma of seemingly contradictory demands of being caught between being an individual and being a member of society.

I believe that *The Human Side of Diabetes* may help resolve the dilemma of wanting to be recognized as a unique individual and of being labeled and treated as a "diabetic." I feel that resolving this dilemma is very important. First, such a resolution can help a person just be a happier person by seeing that labeled people are individuals also. I believe that most of us need to reaffirm or to have reaffirmed that we are a person—not a number, not a cog in an occupational machine, not a faceless consumer, not a label. A celebration of individuality benefits us all.

Second, the resolution of the individual-society dilemma just might help improve the care and treatment of people with diabetes. Those with diabetes and those working with those with diabetes may be better able to treat the "diabetic" because they might recognize that individual human needs exist and that certain responses to the disease may be characteristic of those with the disease or may be a particular response by a single person. Too often people suffer unnecessarily because they think that they are the only one who has ever felt a certain way—such as hating the disease—or done a certain thing—like eating a whole cheesecake as an act of defiance. Too often sincere health-care professionals have dismissed a mood, a response to treatment, or a symptom because it was "typical" of "diabetics." Unless reconsidered as possibly a common occurrence or a unique situation, either the silent suffering or the automatic dismissal could hamper the treatment of the diabetes by affecting the emotional terrain. Such responses might even disguise genuine physical problems and endanger the person's health.

In *The Human Side of Diabetes*, I hope to suggest that the middle ground between living as a label and living in hibernation is beneficial. I also would like to document that the middle ground exists and to indicate how a person might achieve it.

Not unlike many of the people living today, people with diabetes are invisible. For those who have diabetes—patients and their families—and those who treat the disease—doctors, nurses, educators, nutritionists, and others, the disease can result either in stereotypes or hibernation. When one becomes a "diabetic," frequently certain assumptions are made about that person and he or she tends to be treated in certain automatic ways. Likewise people who have diabetes often tend to respond to those who are attempting to help treat the disease by assigning them such labels as "normal," "doctor," "nurse," "nag," or "non-diabetic." The labels and the perfunctory responses they tend to bring about dehumanize everyone involved. As this happens, those with the disease and those treating it tend to retreat—to become closet "diabetics" or distant health-care professionals. They become invisible people.

Diabetes is a complex disease that recently has drawn greater attention from the public and from the medical profession. As the disease has appeared in the households of more and more families and as its complications have been charted and studied more carefully for a longer period of time, medical science has made tremendous strides in improving treatment and curtailing the potentially devastating effects of diabetes. Much has been written about the disease. Refinements have steadily improved the ways and the means for monitoring control, measuring the disease's progress, and for treating it. Greater efforts have been made to improve the patient education programs so that people with diabetes can implement their own improved care. But the fact remains that, despite all of these advancements in the science of the disease, not as much progress is evident in the human applications of this new technology.

I believe that frequently a gap exists between the technology and the individuals who are supposed to be benefiting from it or who are using it.

This book, I hope, will contribute to the closing of that gap. By telling the story of the human side of diabetes from a "diabetic's" perspective, I am striving to demonstrate that neither the "diabetic" nor the "doctor" needs to behave according to a label nor to hibernate when living with or treating diabetes. I have not always known this. In fact, the writing of this book itself happened to occasion most of my discoveries about myself, about diabetes, and about treating diabetes. I have been an invisible person emerging. The benefits of taking the seeming risks in moving away from the safety of labels or of hibernation are enjoyed more and more each day. I would like to share the experience of emerging as well as what I have learned about people, diabetes, and living with (against?) diabetes. I believe that acknowledging the human side of diabetes—opening up to fears and hopes, suggesting approaches and strategies, sharing good and bad experiences—is an essential step towards establishing a genuine attitude for wellness. To really believe that I am human first and "diabetic" second is to live better and to be, I believe, healthier. (In my opinion, acknowledging our humanness can help battle much of what ails us as people in the twentieth century.) To have diabetes does not diminish a person's humanity. I believe that to recognize the unique but shared characteristics of being human and having diabetes can encourage a greater and more effective participation in a therapeutic alliance.

That is the ambitious goal of *The Human Side of Diabetes*. I invite you to join me in attempting to achieve it.

Out of the Closet

For more than three decades, my diabetes and I were in a closet.

I would not tell anyone that I had diabetes. Through elementary school, junior high school, high school, and college, none of my teachers and few of my friends knew I had the disease. Not one of my coaches for football, basketball, wrestling, baseball, or swimming from fourth grade through college intramurals knew. The wrestling coach was kept in the dark about why I couldn't go down another weight class. I don't know how many insulin reactions I tried to "tough out" during football practice while running wind sprints in the hot August sun. My silence permitted uninterrupted strings of erratic meals at a variety of times, unbalanced meals frequently dominated by Cokes and potato chips, and high-stress episodes of hiding in rest rooms while giving myself insulin injections. My refusal to drink beer and "hard liquor" was attributed inaccurately to a reputation for being a "goody-goody" and may have resulted in my not being invited to many parties.

Rather than reveal my secret, I weighed carefully every situation from age nine on. When I dated, I never hinted of a disease that would be with me throughout my life. Job applications always were marked "excellent" in the health spaces. Part-time or full-time employers—whether an armature factory, a city parks department, a finance company, the telephone company, or a variety of educational institutions—were never informed.

But it was more than not telling people that I had diabetes. I worked hard at denying that I had the disease. First, I just gave myself an injection in the morning and forgot it all. I ate and drank what was available. I did not check my sugar levels. I avoided doctors, dentists, or anyone who had ever been near a medical school. I would not read anything about diabetes and refused to talk about it as a disease. I winced when loved ones asked, "How are you feel ing?" or "How have you been?" I did not think about the future.

Second, I denied my diabetes by insisting on demonstrating that I could not only do what others could do, but also more. I pushed myself physically to dangerous extremes just to show that I could "cut it." Whether at work or play, I always tried to do it all. "Diabetes? What diabetes?" Many times I would play three sets of tennis in the morning, ride ten miles on a bicycle in the afternoon, and play racquetball that night. Work days—especially early in my career—frequently started at 7:00 A.M. and ended at 2:00 or 3:00 o'clock the next morning. Moonlighting jobs often included loading and unloading eighteen-wheeler tractor trailers for household moves, digging by hand drain fields for septic tanks, and painting house exteriors in the middle of July. I would not tolerate any suggestion of fatigue or anyone asking me if I were "okay." In my efforts to deny my diabetes, I would not allow myself to be human with human limitations. I reacted bitterly to any evidence of my limitations—even limitations that someone without diabetes would have. I was never tired, thirsty, nor sore; I always was ready to go, strong enough to lift anything, and eager to take on any job.

But, even though I did not tell people that I had diabetes and acted as if I didn't have it, the disease would not disappear. Missed meals, overexertion, and unchanged insulin dosages frequently resulted in insulin reactions, exhaustion, and dehydration. Diabetes also lurked forever in my mind. Too many times I had been told of the price of denial. I kept thinking about having to pay that price. What was coming? How long did I have?Ironically, my body kept fooling me—before I knew it I was 16, then 21, then 30, then 35, and even 40! The pressure built with each birthday. To me, each birthday marked the approach of the time that I would have to make the payment on that terrible debt.

The pressure seemed to get so incredible that, upon the insistence and guidance of a dear friend who was a psychiatric nurse, I decided to check out the damage. With Alberta's persistent arm twisting, I forced myself to see a diabetes nurse specialist who persuaded me to see a doctor who persuaded me to check into a hospital for a week. It was this visit to the hospital which occasioned my emergence and that of my diabetes from the closet.

Because of that hospital visit, I met a bunch of delightful people. Some were fellow patients in the hospital because of their diabetes. Because we all were on a special diabetes unit, we shared something—the disease—which made it easier for us to get to know each other. Once that happened we were eager to keep in touch after we were out of the unit. I met Jack—a tough young news and sports cameraman for a local television station. As "roomies" in the hospital, we shared war stories about sports and diabetes. I met Dawne, a perky sophomore in college who—when on the "outside"—was majoring in psychology while single-handedly running the university's student union. I met Bruce—a 26-year-old policeman devoted to athletics, body building, hunting, and fishing.

Some other delightful people who had diabetes were introduced to me while they were acting on behalf of a diabetes support group. Once introduced to the support group idea while on the unit, I was persuaded to give one of their monthly meetings a try. At that first meeting, I met Maggie—a ball of fire with a sharp tongue, a true wit, and a heart of gold who is at home on the archery range, in the library, or around the medical laboratory. I met Buster—a rough-and-tough rancher who carries a gun and makes John Wayne look like a caricature. I met Georgianna—a fashion plate manager of an area department store whose smile outshines her wardrobe. I met Dick—a veteran fire chief who would do anything he could to protect others from fires. Buster served as leader of the group while Maggie took care of the paperwork, Georgianna helped with the programming, and Dick did "whatever had to be done."

While each of these people were of different ages, educational backgrounds, cultural heritages, and occupations, they were friendly, vigorous, and fun to be with. Each also happened to have diabetes. They were not in any closet. In fact, a few of them—such as Maggie, Buster, and Georgianna—were downright outspoken about their being people who just happened to have diabetes.

They don't know it, but they brought me out of *my* closet. They did not lecture about being "nearly normal," nor parade about proclaiming how wonderfully they had adjusted, nor promise the delights of bringing one's diabetes out into the open. They were friends. They just lived their lives and shared their lives. Over cans of diet soda, Maggie talked about teaching and living one-on-one. Buster loved giving barbecues on his cattle ranch. Always dressed to the teeth, Georgianna talked freely at the support group meetings about her insulin pump and its role in her career. They were friends who happen to have diabetes. But their models were enough. They showed me how life could be out of the closet.

Sometimes I think they unintentionally may have created a monster. Not only have I told those close to me at home, work, or play that I have diabetes, but also I have been telling complete strangers. I have not only been making concessions to the diabetes, but I also have been insisting upon them and have not been shy about explaining to others why the concessions are important to me. I even have given lectures and participated in support group discussions—telling anyone who might listen to my own story about hiding in the closet with my diabetes.

The results seem to have made it worthwhile. By coming out, I have been able to learn that I am not alone. Many admit to sharing the same sorts of feelings and experiences. The sense of being a part of a community has made it all worthwhile. I no longer feel entirely like some sort of weirdo. I am not so different; I am not so alone. Diabetes seems a lot less intimidating.

Furthermore, the sharing of feelings and experiences has been very educational—it has taught me a great deal about the tricks of coping and of living with the disease. When a few of us talk sometimes, between us we are utilizing over one hundred years' worth of experience with diet, insulin, exercise, and the medical profession. It is rare when a new situation comes up; inevitably someone has been there before!

With this informal education has come a great deal of relief. I find that I have been worrying about "imminent disasters" which probably will never occur. For example, I used to believe that my children had more than a 50% chance of developing diabetes. New research, my friends informed me, reveals that the actual odds are less than 5%! Things which had seemed to be the mysterious province of the medical profession in its white magical coats have turned out to be accessible to anyone living with diabetes. Blood glucose monitoring no longer had to be an expensive trip to the laboratory or doctor's office. Anyone could change insulin dosages: a doctor's permission was not necessary. More than one type of insulin or diet existed. Once out of the closet, my life with diabetes turned out to be much more enlightened than it had been for over three decades.

Also, by coming out of the closet, I have had some impact on others who have also been lingering alone in despair and fear. After my hospital stay, I returned to the classroom at the university, and in a few months I had discovered that four of my students, an employee in the bookstore, a daughter of a secretary in the education department, and a niece of a good friend in the registrar's office were all struggling with diabetes. Soon we were sharing war stories, recommending doctors, and exchanging encouragement. In some cases, the sharing of the diabetes serves only as an icebreaker. Once total strangers or mere acquaintances, some of us have become good friends after getting to know each other because we shared the disease.

In short, a whole new world has opened to me since I was coaxed out of the closet with my diabetes.

Enlightenment

Judy looked up from her counted cross-stitch one night and quietly stated, "You know, for a person with about 400 years of formal education, you're not very bright."

"Oh, yeah?" I muttered. "Give me a for-instance." I, not being very bright, attributed her subsequent silence to the lack of evidence.

"Come on, just one example, that's all—just one," I pressed. "Well? Why am I so dumb?"

My refusal to let her remark slide showed she was correct.

My wife of decades smiled and asked, "What have you been doing for the last 30 minutes?"

"So? What does that matter? It's a free country. I'm entitled to my opinions."

I had been moaning and groaning about doctors, diabetes, heart disease, diets, and all the other fertilizer that "sure screws up a normal life." That day I had been to see a local physician about an upper-respiratory infection and had gotten a perfunctory lecture on diabetes—focused on its complications—and a urine test. The lecture was gloomy black; the urine turned bright orange. That evening I moaned, groaned, and complained.

"Why don't you do something about it?" she inquired.

"The doctors in this town flunked out of veterinary school!" I snapped. "They're idiots!"

"If a person with 400 years of formal education was unhappy with something in one town, what might he consider?"

"That's easy for you to say!" I roared as I stomped out of the room.

Not very bright.

As usual, Judy was right. I was nearly paralyzed by my fears, my ignorance, and my distrust of the medical care in the small town we had lived in for more than a decade. I hadn't been to a doctor for diabetes in over 11 years. I didn't go because I was sure I was on the edge of a medical disaster.

After several more months of careful consideration—and some severe strong-arm tactics by those who loved me—I did "the right thing." (It actually required very little of my academic training to find a distinctive diabetes care unit in a city only 35 miles away.)

The six days in the hospital were truly enlightening. I learned I wasn't nearly as bad off medically as I had feared. I learned I was in the dark ages about diabetes care. The health-care team taught me about the changes in treatments and attitudes, and showed me how to take care of myself. No one in the hospital threatened me; there were no urine sugar tests; food wasn't treated as an enemy; having diabetes wasn't the end of the world. I came home with a mountain of new information, new procedures, and a seemingly new perception of myself and diabetes care.

However, after being back in our small town for some time, I found myself failing to use much of my new medical education or any of my academic training. The fear, guilt, and despair returned. I now "knew a lot about diabetes," but sometimes I didn't feel so super and the glucose monitoring wasn't documenting the exquisite results I expected. Why was my blood glucose over 200? I should be doing better: the guilt returned. Clearly, there was more to this disease than I had imagined. More and more reading turned up few substantial insights: the old despair began to dim my newfound bright future. I felt like a "diabetic-in-exile." The experts were miles away busy with their important work with patients in the hospital who really needed their help. I didn't want to, but I slipped back in to my growing fears and then gave in to my instincts for isolation. As the gloom seeped in, the attention to the diet, the exercise, and the monitoring slipped.

I returned to moaning and groaning about "that damn diabetes," complaining "I don't know what to do," and whining about feeling "so alone."

Judy was working on another cross-stitch project, but her doubts about my intelligence sounded familiar.

"You know, for a person with about 400 years of formal education, you're not very bright."

"What? What? What should I do?" Even I was bright enough to recognize the futility of resisting her counter cross-stitch logic.

"Why don't you do something?"

"What? What? What should I do?"

"What do you need?"

"Help. I need help!"

"Get it then."

"Where? There's no one in this town. . . ." The echo was loud and clear. After a few days of hoping all of my problems would go away, I called the diabetes nurse specialist at the unit late one afternoon, when the pace at the hospital is less frantic.

Beth listened to my moans and groans, snorts and screams. Once I sensed her willingness to listen, I was unable to refrain from expressing my feelings of ignorance and fear and my sense of isolation. When I collapsed into exhausted silence, Beth offered some suggestions for modifying the insulin dosages ("Remember, we set up your plan in the hospital. Now, you are living in less than ideal circumstances, and some tinkering needs to be done.") and indicated that I was doing better than I gave myself credit for.

"Why don't you come to a party that Maggie and Buster are giving this weekend?"

"Hmm . . . aww . . . well . . . ah . . . okay . . . I guess so." I didn't have the heart—after her listening to me for over 20 minutes—to repeat my ingrained aversion to parties given by people with diabetes for people with diabetes.

"Great. See you Saturday, and don't hesitate to call me if you're having any problems or just want to talk."

Hanging up, I couldn't believe I'd agreed to go to a diabetes support group party. For months I had ignored written invitations, personal charm, and veiled threats ("Don't knock my parties until you've tried them."). I didn't know why: the group was organized by and for people with diabetes; it was independent of any hospital or physician; its primary goal was social support.

That Saturday wasn't nearly as bad as I had expected. In fact, if the truth be known, I had a great time! Once I stopped taking "How are you doing?" as a personal accusation, I noticed that this so-called support group meeting was a regular party. Table upon table was laden with all sorts of food—some healthy, some not-so-healthy, some downright sinful. Individuals, families, friends, and strangers were enjoying themselves: talking, riding horses, swimming, playing volleyball and softball, and just hanging out. They seemed like regular people. They talked about sports, languished in their day off, and teased each other. Pretty soon I stopped trying to figure out which member in each family or group was the one with diabetes. When diabetes did come up, these people were very comfortable with it as a topic of conversation. They were easy on themselves as well as those around them. They were pleasant people.

As we ate, drank, played, and compared notes on kids, taxes, the economy, and traffic in a rapidly growing Florida, I discovered myself having a good time. I felt different. I didn't feel alone. I didn't feel like the only victim of diabetes in a dark universe. I somehow sensed that living did not require my knowing all there was to know about diabetes. I felt good. I experienced a sense of hope. It was fun being a person having a good time on a Saturday. It was fun having fun.

As I drove home, I knew I wasn't cured of diabetes. I knew that my fear, ignorance, and despair were not gone forever. The battle was not over. But I was happy. I didn't feel so alone. As the cars whizzed by me on the interstate highway, I grinned with the feeling that the people in those cars and I were of the same species. I just happen to have diabetes.

Maybe they did too. If they did, I knew they could call an expert at the hospital if they needed help. If they did, I knew of a group of people—some who may have diabetes—who were more than willing to give a party, to meet monthly for a bull session, or to organize educational programs about living with diabetes.

For a guy with more than 400 years of formal education, I have learned quite a bit lately. I feel brighter.

50 Miles to the Light

For years, I had been going to a local doctor who specialized in internal medicine. The doctor routinely recommended tighter control of the diabetes, but provided little insight on how to attain it. He regularly ordered fasting blood sugars and chided me regardless of the result. He dispensed the same pre-fabricated diet sheets with each visit. On one occasion, he even told me that my insulin reactions were imaginary and instructed me to go get a blood sugar test the next time I thought I was low. (I did, in fact, drive the seven miles to the hospital while suffering with one of my "imaginary" insulin reactions to record a 56 blood sugar, well below the normal 80-120 range.) The insulin dosages were never changed. My control did not improve, but I never pressed the doctor for more information on how to deal with the disease more effectively. Then this doctor left town to retrain as a cardiac specialist.

A new internal medicine specialist came to town. He seemed more aggressive about dealing with diabetes, but he was not very interested in diet or in changing the insulin dosages. His nurse did blood sugars in the office with a refectance meter, and the doctor pushed me to purchase my own machine. (Unfortunately the doctor arranged the purchase of a machine that he had never used and without seeming to know that other machines were available that were easier to use and cheaper.) Frequently the nurse would instruct me about insulin injections and Clinitest urine testing. I went to the new doctor for three years. I tried the "new" ideas. The machine was difficult to use; the monitoring results were not translated into changes in the handling of my disease; the doctor seemed at a loss for what to do next. I lost confidence in the new ideas and the internist. So, I stopped seeing this doctor and did not go to another one for several years.

Other people with diabetes were not as passive about their health care as I was. Unsatisfied with the kind of care I had been receiving, they sought better, more up-to-date, and more personal treatment. They were willing to drive 50 miles to appointments if necessary. They talked about new and varied treatments for diabetes they were learning about and using. They were going to nurses and doctors who specialized in diabetes and who worked with diabetes programs and diabetes care units in hospitals. Those actively participating in their own diabetes care talked enthusiastically about new research findings, better treatment techniques, and how they came to adopt their positive attitudes and a sense of hope.

The possibility of hope stirred me to some tentative action. One day, with strong encouragement from a friend, I managed an introductory visit with a diabetes nurse specialist. A few weeks later, I dared to walk through a diabetes care unit. Surviving the visit and hours of persuasion, I finally agreed to make an appointment with an endocrinologist specializing in diabetes. During the first office visit, the physician suggested that diabetes care was a case of making choices. He convinced me that for a treatment program to work it must suit the life of the person with diabetes. A week later, I drove the 50 miles to check into a diabetes care unit for a complete medical evaluation and a patient education program.

As my stay in the unit progressed, I felt like I was emerging from a dark cell into bright sunlight.

First of all, I learned that diabetes was a much more complex disease than my small-town doctors had led me to believe.

Up-to-date information offered more and more comfort. There were more insulins from several companies than I could have ever dreamed. Besides the pork and beef insulins I had been using without question, there were purified pork and beef as well as synthetic human insulins. Some of the purified insulins were more pure than others. The synthetic insulins so resembled natural human insulin that they were absorbed better and apparently did not result in the patient's body producing antibodies to resist the presence and work of the "foreign" substances. Plus there were insulin pumps for those who were insulin-dependent. Rather than taking frequent shots, a person with diabetes could wear a small, light machine that is programmed to provide insulin in specific amounts at prescribed times through an injection site. I also learned about a wide variety of pills for those with late-onset diabetes (Type II) to take to lower their blood glucose.

Home glucose monitoring, considered a necessity rather than a convenience or a luxury, was now to be done several times a day. A wide array of monitoring devices were available. By using the glucose monitoring and working with the health-care professionals, many people develop a sliding scale for their insulin dosages. They adjust their insulin dosages with each testing of the blood sugar. Multiple insulin injections a day had become commonplace.

My stay at the unit also showed me that carbohydrates were not the enemy. Vegetarian or high fiber diets were not fads. Eating was done five times a day.

Factors other than insulin, food, and exercise had been discovered to affect blood glucose levels. Stress had been discovered to act like chocolate ice cream while humor serves as exercise.

All sorts of equipment and procedures now existed to help develop in-depth evaluations of a patient's physical condition. Treatments had been developed to combat the complications associated with diabetes.

The second focus that helped me move from the dark and into the light was the unit's focus on teaching diabetes self-care. Diabetes patient education was as important as primary medical care. The dominant attitude was that the person with diabetes and his or her family were the most important people in the treatment of the disease. Rather than a treatment program which centered on directives from the medical "gods-on-high," the aim now was for the patient to decide what to do. I was taught what choices were available and the possible significance of each decision, but I had to make the choice. For effective self-care, I was encouraged to become actively involved in my diabetes care. Furthermore, I learned that I needed to constantly review and evaluate what the medical team and I were doing. And during my stay, I was given ample opportunity to practice this new concept of self-care.

I felt as if I had been released from shackles that had been holding me in a prison. I felt much freer, like my life and control of my life had been returned to me.

As I left the diabetes care unit to drive the 50 miles back home, the journey seemed so short. It seemed such an easy trip in a sunny, hopeful world. I felt great and was home with Judy, Eric, and Bryan before I knew it. I chided myself for not acting sooner on my lack of faith in the hometown physicians. I asked the idiot living inside my body a few pointed questions: Why had I allowed myself to swallow my discomfort with and anxieties about the medical care I had been receiving? Why had I been so slow to respond to others' advice to check out what other medical professionals had to offer? What had I to lose by admitting that doctors and nurses are human and can be as imperfect as anyone? Why couldn't I admit that not everyone might be up-to-date in diabetes research and care? Why had I clung to my dark fears for so long?

Fifty miles seemed such a short distance to travel to move into the light.

Freed by the Philmont Scout Ranch

I NEVER HAVE BEEN sure whether Dad and Mom knew what they were doing or whether it was just a stroke of good fortune. But, whatever the cause, I know that the events they encouraged resulted in a major turning point in my life.

One cold February evening I returned from my Boy Scout troop meeting warmed with enthusiasm. The Scoutmaster had made a short presentation about the Philmont Scout Ranch in New Mexico. His description of the adventurous trip across country, the strenuous backpacking, the primitive camping, and the risky mountain climbing would have fired up the imagination of even the greenest of tenderfoots. As a fourteen-year-old second-class Scout, I was pretty excited as I repeated to my parents the Scoutmaster's marvelous sales pitch for the three-week adventure.

My parents were surprised. Although I had played Little League baseball, delivered the Philadelphia *Bulletin*, mowed lawns, and done the usual stuff as a kid, I had hung fairly close to home. Having had diabetes for about five years, I had been carefully watched and had grown more and more self-conscious as a "diabetic." Oh, I had gone to the Elliot P. Joslin Diabetic Camp for Children for two summers, but everyone there had diabetes and was the object of some sort of research. When my father had had his heart attacks, I had been the only child to go with my mother to the various hospitals in the various cities. Responsibilities for the day-to-day management of my diabetes had not been completely assumed by my parents, but—to be sure—Mom had handled the diet and the daily injections more often than I had. While not totally dependent, I certainly was not independent.

My parents were subtle, but their questions about the Philmont trip quickly came to the point.

Questions about cost, itinerary, length, and transportation were soon followed with more direct inquiries.

"Who would be going with you?"

"Do you think you could handle yourself?"

"Would you watch your diet?"

"What about your injections? Would you be able to give your-self your shot for three weeks straight? Will you be willing to give yourself your shots? Can you take enough insulin and needles with you?"

"Do you think someone with diabetes would be allowed or should be allowed to go on the trip?"

"Are you willing to take responsibility for the diabetes?"

"Will you take care of yourself?"

"Do you think you can do it alone?"

"Do you want to do it?"

The answers about the trip's details came easily; the answers about my managing my own diabetes did not come as readily. I had not thought about my diabetes. When I did, I found that I was not too confident and less enthusiastic about the trip.

Diet? Sugar monitoring? Injections? Insulin reactions? All that stuff? No, I had not thought much about diabetes in connection with Philmont. The more I did, the more I began to hesitate. An animated dialogue between skeptical parents and enthusiastic Boy Scout turned into questions alternating with "hmm's" and "aahh's" and "well, I don't know's."

But I had shot off my mouth and felt compelled to follow through. I would send off for the brochure with the full information and then back off. I vowed I would be more circumspect the next time.

Dad did not wait for the brochure. Every day he would talk about Philmont and would dream out loud about the joys of back-packing and camping. Each day he seemed to get more enthusiastic about Philmont. By the time the colorful brochure arrived, he had offered to pay half of the cost.

The brochure was, indeed, enticing. Colorful photographs and purple prose promised an exciting cross-country bus trip and showed majestic mountains and sparkling streams. It hinted at un-specified adventures; it talked of comraderie, manhood, and self-sufficiency. Philmont sounded great, but my parents' questions had raised the issue of how willing I was to "rough it" or, for that mat-ter, to take full responsibility for my life and my diabetes.

I ended up going anyway. I went because it sounded like fun and because my parents had just assumed I would—not because I had made some sort of monumental decision to become more responsible for myself and my diabetes.

As 23 Boy Scouts and four leaders headed from New Jersey by bus towards New Mexico, I privately tested and gave myself injections. Only the adult leaders knew of my diabetes. The only worries involved with the side trips to the Indianapolis Speedway, Dodge City, the Air Force Academy, Denver, and a Navaho reservation were how to ration my souvenir money.

But, when we hit the Philmont Scout Ranch, I began to tense up. The "roughing it" portion of the trip had arrived: soon I would be out in the mountains, cut off from any civilization, and fully responsible for myself as we hiked 10 to 15 miles a day. We would carry everything—food, clothing, tents, and medications—on our backs. We would be on our own.

After a day of orientation, expedition 804-E left the base camp and headed into the Rocky Mountains. Two weeks later, 22 advanced Scouts and one second-class Scout with diabetes emerged triumphantly. Oh, our adventure had not been without its tribulations. One guy had nearly drowned; another had suffered from smoke inhalation; a leader had broken his arm mountain climbing.

I even had my episodes. Early in the trip, my fellow Scouts were curious about my refusal to let anyone carry one particular satchel (the one with the syringes, needles, insulins, and antibiotics). But once on the trail, others teased me about disappearing into the tent just before breakfast (I was giving myself my injections). Once I told them I had diabetes and had to take shots they were less awkward around me. In a short time, I was one of the guys. I didn't bring up my diabetes, and it rarely was an issue for anyone but me on the trip.

Sometimes the episodes were more serious. One day—due to a downpour—my group was late getting dinner ready. Because the meal was late, my blood sugar got too low. Unfortunately, because we were rushing to feed the howling mob, I did not recognize the early symptoms of an insulin reaction. I got into a fight with my tent mate George. We remained cool to each other for some time. I was unable to explain adequately the effects of a very low blood sugar. ("Isn't low sugar what you want?")

On another occasion, I was a part of a group of 10 Scouts who had gotten lost and separated from the food. We missed the noon meal. By mid-afternoon, I could feel a severe insulin reaction coming on, but did not have any simple sugars with me to counteract it. I alerted the group. We tried to find our way to the next camp and the food, but I passed out. Yogi, a fellow Scout, ran on to bring back first aid and food. After I recovered from the reaction and regained consciousness, I was embarrassed by my "weakness" and chagrined at what I had made Yogi go through. It was a few days on the trail before I finally relaxed and stopped worrying about a recurrence. (Carrying half a dozen chocolate bars in my drug satchel also helped reduce my fear.)

Despite the mishaps, the Scouts from the Gloucester-Salem Council of New Jersey came out of the Rocky Mountains unbeaten and unbowed. To a person—including the one with diabetes—we proclaimed the trip, "Great!"

I had learned so much about walking 15 miles a day with a full pack. Reading maps and nature, I had climbed the Rocky Mountains and crossed beautiful, ice-cold rivers and streams. Taking pride in the rigorous labors—the walking, the climbing, the camping, the cooking, and the sometimes hostile weather—I had wrestled with stubborn mules—human as well as animal. I had had many chances to cook meals for over two dozen people at one time, to share the successes as well as the failures over the campfire, and to enjoy the sense of growing brotherhood. Each warm day and cool night was a glorious event.

For me, life had taken on a new texture.

I returned to my sophomore year of high school a new person—physically and emotionally. Strong and in excellent condition, I went out for varsity football for the first time ever. In fact, I tried out for offensive guard—at 135 pounds—because I knew that, even with the diabetes, I could run, block, and tackle with my peers. Hadn't I kept up with 22 trained Scouts for two weeks in the New Mexico mountains? I also was elected Student Council vice-president. Diabetes hadn't inhibited me from being a leader among 27 boys and men trained and experienced in leadership. How could it be any different in a rather tame high school? My whole life took on new dimensions socially and academically. If I could handle drugs, injections, diet, exercise, and the rigors of life in the wilderness, living with diabetes in civilization no longer seemed that big a deal.

I was enjoying my heightened sense of self. I felt more capable physically. I seemed more attuned to the world around me—the na-ture, the people, the pace, the pleasures, and the pains.

The Philmont trip provided a crucial turning point in my life.

Because I did have diabetes and had had a successful—although frequently trying—experience at Philmont, I felt suddenly free. I no longer felt like a "diabetic." I had gone into the wilderness sym-bolically loaded down with the burdens of the disease. I came out with the diabetes, but with a diminished sense of its burden. My body was muscled, tanned, and healthy. It had met very real chal-lenges. It had survived Philmont. I was convinced that it could sur-vive other things and meet other challenges. I was convinced that living could be primary in my life and that the diabetes could be secondary—if not incidental—to it. I felt like any other human be-ing. I felt free.

Badges of Courage

Ever since I was a little tyke, everyone urged me to have some sort of identification card in my wallet or some sort of jewelry that announced that I had diabetes. They pointed to the possibilities of my falling victim to an insulin reaction or lapsing into coma or other ominous, unspecified catastrophes.

"How would people know what to do," they warned, "if you passed out in public or were so disoriented that you couldn't provide vital information? How would people know to call a doctor or to take you to the hospital? You should wear some ID."

Not me! I was not going to announce that I have diabetes. No way. While I was not too excited about people knowing that I had diabetes, why would I want to advertise it with a necklace or a bracelet that dangles from my body? What if someone were to go into my wallet? My secret would be out. Diabetes was *my* private business.

But, as time went by and I had been through a few rough insulin reactions, I submitted to the pressure. I didn't go for the jewelry; I filled out a card with my name, address, and phone number; my doctor's name, address, and phone number; and my usual insulin dosage. The card didn't cost anything and could be hid discreetly in my wallet. That free paper card quickly wore out and was replaced only when another free card was available.

After 28 years of "discreet identification," I am now wearing a necklace that identifies me as a "diabetic." (I am not delighted with that label.) No catastrophe occasioned this radical shift from my refusal to advertise that I had diabetes. It occurred for two reasons.

First, I stopped being ashamed of having diabetes. As I came out of the closet, I worked on being less self-conscious about the disease. As I became more aware of the fact that diabetes was not a punishment for something I had or had not done, I did not see the jewelry as some sort of mark of Cain. As I demonstrated more and more that I could do just about anything I set out to do, I was more willing to acknowledge that I had a chronic disease. As I saw that many, many very decent people happen to have the disease, I became more willing to be seen as one of them. They wore their jewelry and were not embarrassed or shy about it. Why should I be?

Second, while at a support group meeting of people with diabetes and of health-care professionals, a deputy sheriff who happen to have diabetes told us that emergency personnel such as firemen, paramedics, and police were not allowed to go into the wallets of people they were trying to help. The victim had to give them permission—which is fairly difficult when the victim is unconscious!

Since I had started being more careful about controlling my sugars—and therefore was more likely to be a victim of insulin reactions—I bought a cheap medical alert necklace. What is even more important is that I actually wear it!

But it was not easy. I was very self-conscious, especially when I had my shirt off for swimming or fishing. I found myself fiddling with it and actually drawing attention to it by mistake. Sometimes I just forgot to put it on before leaving the house for the day. (I had never worn any jewelry my whole life until I got married, and Judy insisted that if I wished to remain alive I'd better keep the ring on.) Sometimes I just forgot it on purpose. There were a million reasons: it'll get in the way; I won't need it; it doesn't go with my outfit.

A dear friend came to my rescue by giving me a good luck piece. The attractive piece of jewelry could be worn anywhere, but since I already had on the medical identification necklace I just slipped the good luck piece onto the same chain. So I now have to wear the identification necklace: how could I play cards or drive my car or play tennis or face the cruel world without my good luck piece—which just so happens to be attached to the medical alert piece? I now wear my good luck piece and my medical alert jewelry every day together.

Fortunately, my history with medical identification jewelry goes beyond my submission to pressure or the trickery of behavior modification. Wearing the jewelry has become a symbolic act. In the last few years, I have met a lot of people who happen to have diabetes. They are, on the whole, extremely pleasant people who know how to live. Most significant, however, is that they are not embarrassed about having diabetes. They do not seem ashamed of having the disease. They are not "closet diabetics." They wear their medical identification jewelry and they wear it proudly. Some, in fact, go to great lengths to make the jewelry special and conspicuous. One wears an elaborate gold medallion around her neck; another had a special bracelet made for him.

Their example has served me well. As I have learned more about diabetes and have decided to challenge the disease rather than succumb to it passively, I have tried to imitate what I believe to be their courage. Their openness with their jewelry represents their open courage about their diabetes. They are bold; they are forthright.

As I wear my necklace, I try to wear it as they do—a badge of courage.

PART II

Day-to-Day

"His Life is Over!"

MANY YEARS AGO, a young boy's family learned that the nine-year-old had diabetes. The family's responses were unfortunate.

"My God, diabetic! Oh, no!"

"He'll never lead a normal life."

"Why us? Why us? It isn't fair!"

"His life is over!"

These heartfelt outcries reflected the family's genuine love for the boy and anguish over the news. But, to a young boy who didn't understand that, these initial, unguarded outbursts provided early ominous cues.

More recently, a twenty-five-year-old police officer was diagnosed as having Type-I (insulin-dependent) diabetes. Although much more is now known about living with diabetes and no one had suggested that his life was over, despair also characterized this recent introduction to the disease. The officer provided it himself. Despair and fear dominated his every question.

"Can I still be a cop? Will I be able to make detective?"

"Will I be able to hunt and fish?"

"Will I be able to run, lift weights, body build, play ball, or do any of the things I love?"

"Should I marry?"

"Should I have children?"

"What does this mean to my life? Is my life over?"

If left unanswered, the nine-year-old's experiences and the twenty-five-year-old's questions can allow anxieties to grow in such a way as to enclose and then, perhaps, to paralyze each person's life.

As that nine-year-old, I was to go on for 28 years fighting like mad to disprove my family's outbursts. Determined to be "normal," I tried to deny that I had diabetes. I did what I pleased. I went out of my way to eat what I was told I shouldn't. I ignored warnings and precautions. I avoided doctors. I threw myself into activities with a grimness which belied my youth. I lived each day as if it were my last.

But I never forgot that my "life was over" at age nine. My family's pessimistic outbursts stayed with me and haunted me. No matter how hard I tried, my fears could not be ignored. An ominous cloud hung over my life as I waited for the disasters my family had assured me would come. I found no reason for working on controlling the diabetes.

"What's the use?" I would think, as I recalled over and over again my parents' emotional "His life is over." To this day, I still am trying to overcome their "death sentence."

In contrast, the twenty-five-year-old police officer had an opportunity to have his questions answered. He is certain that the early opportunity to discuss his questions had an important impact on how he initially responded to living with his diabetes.

Because of my experience with diabetes and of my growing awareness of how my parents' reaction to my diagnosis had influenced me, I had offered to talk with anyone who might want an "insider's" view of the disease. One day a diabetes unit's head nurse called and asked me to drop in at the hospital and chat with Bruce, the police officer. The officer and I talked primarily about my life. We started with "war" stories about my high school and college careers playing football, basketball, tennis, and baseball and participating in swimming and wrestling. We then joked about my middle-aged departure from contact sports to just tennis, racquetball, and bicycling. We talked about dating, my marriage, and my two healthy sons. The officer was curious about the other things I had been able to do: paint houses, dig septic tank drain fields, build additions upon houses, and work with a long-haul truck driver. Neither of us would reveal our favorite fishing holes. The officer discovered himself having a "normal" conversation.

We even got around to talking about diabetes. The newly-diagnosed interrogated me about everything from exercise, diet, and complications to the psychological, emotional, and personal aspects of trying to live with the disease. Not all the news was good. He took the risk of asking the hard questions, and I responded to his courage by being as honest as possible. I kept reminding him I didn't know everything and my experiences might not always be typical. But we grew more comfortable with each other and with talking about diabetes.

I left with hope that Bruce would not suffer as I had with the long and often torturous adjustment period that can come with diabetes and with the struggles to discover how his life will be affected. My hope seemed to have some basis. Bruce had started to take deep breaths; his eyes suggested that some of his fear had diminished. Reports are that, when he left the hospital, he departed with intentions of resuming his life as it was and of living with his diabetes.

People newly-diagnosed with diabetes should be careful about investing too much in how they are told about the disease and what they are told initially. Remember that people are emotional and frequently have a difficult time telling others bad news. We also are not very good at getting bad news.

As our two separate histories suggest, a person's initiation into diabetes can be crucial. What is said, how it is done, when it is done, and who does it may dictate the newly diagnosed person's (and the family's) attitude toward his/her life and the diabetes.

If you have diabetes, try not to be too influenced by how you were told that you have the disease.

If you are telling people they have diabetes, be careful how you tell them.

If you know people who have been recently diagnosed, be careful how you react to the news.

Misinformation—or information given while under emotional distress—can endanger the credibility of any information provided later. Uncontrolled fear, anger, or despair while communicating the news can generate the same emotions in those hearing the news. Distraught family members may make the person with diabetes feel guilty or hopeless. Indifference or disinterest may make the person with the chronic disease feel alone or ashamed because he or she is afraid. Strangers carrying the news may not be the best messengers. The newly diagnosed should not be allowed to feel alone with the disease or that the disease is insignificant or "just a common occurrence" or "could be worse." While the doctor or nurse may have seen hundreds of cases of diabetes, it is that person's only case.

People who are familiar with diabetes and care about those who have it make excellent messengers. Those who are not health-care professionals may be even better. Doctors or nurses can be seen as outsiders if they do not have diabetes themselves. The perfect team, perhaps, would be a physician who specializes in diabetes, a family member who has been informed about the disease and about the importance of how he/she reacts, and a person with diabetes who can speak from experience and can identify with the newly diagnosed.

Giving the news of diagnosed diabetes to the person with the disease can be a crucial stage in establishing his or her relationship with the disease, the family, and the health-care professionals. Rapid-fire questions will come, wild emotions will run, and attitudes toward the disease will be set. Anyone involved with the process should know that it all can happen and that it is important.

Those of us who already have been told we have diabetes and have been told in a less-than-ideal way should try to remember not to take the "botched job" to heart.

Our lives are not over.

Taking Shots

"How can you stand taking shots?!?"

"I couldn't bear to take injections every day."

"It's awful that you have to stab yourself every day."

"Does it hurt?"

"Can't you take the pills?"

Such are the usual remarks by the public when they learn that I have insulin-dependent diabetes. Occasionally, I have taken perverse pleasure in replying to such remarks about injections with "What's the alternative?" "I enjoy the excruciating pain," "I prefer the needle to having to swallow a tablet," and "Sure, I gave up injections for a while, but I died." I even have been known to torture unthinking strangers by getting up from a card game and saying, "Well, it's time for that cold shaft of steel" or "I wonder if that needle will bounce today" or "It's time to shoot up!"

The truth about insulin injections for me is that they have been part of a repeating pattern of fear and relief throughout my life.

The first experience with this pattern occurred when I was diagnosed at age nine as having insulin-dependent or Type I diabetes. My father had said in a horrified voice, "My God, he'll have to take shots his whole life!" As a nine-year-old, I quickly developed wild visions of a tortured life of painful injections. I imagined two-foot needles being driven into my thin, frail body as they held me down.

Two days later, when I got to the Joslin Clinic in Boston, anything seemed preferable to insulin injections. As the nurse approached with that first shot, I tensed for a fight. Not me, I wasn't going to be hooked on a life of needles. She slipped it in. I felt better than I had for weeks. Ah, what relief! I did not feel a thing. The shot hadn't hurt. Then fifteen minutes later, the insulin began to have its effect.

The second experience of developing severe apprehensions and then relief associated with injections took place soon after the origi nal one. The day after that first shot, under the guidance of the Joslin Clinic, I checked into the New England Deaconness Hospital for treatment and patient education. After about two days, a nurse informed my parents that they were to start giving me my insulin injections. They nodded with grim determination, and I nearly passed out. I loved them dearly, but I wasn't going to subject myself to the clumsy paws of a nonmedical person for my shots—even if they were my parents. For a whole day they practiced on grapefruit. Each time they stabbed that poor round, yellow fruit I could not help but notice the discrepancy between the size of that citrus and my skinny arms. As the appointed time approached, I grew more and more tense and more and more fervent in my prayers that the next day would be delayed.

But come it did. I snarled as my father prefaced his first attempt with the age-old parental cliché about how this was going to hurt him more than it would me. We all had grim faces as his rookie hand tentatively did its duty. "Not bad," I thought as I mustered a small smile. Mom and Dad went into handsprings of joy. They must have been terrified that I was going to burst out in tears. My smile broadened and my thoughts turned into voiced praise as my parents became more experienced and therefore more confident. Ah, what relief!

But there was little time to rest. Two days later the nurse informed me that I would be giving myself some of my shots while I was in the hospital. I grabbed the grapefruit. I practiced and practiced, grasping that suffering yellow ball of fruit and thrusting in the needle over and over. I followed the nurse's instructions very carefully. Precise, short, swift strokes. Over and over, hour after hour. The fated morning arrived, but my confidence did not. I loaded the syringe. I swiped my skin clean with alcohol. But I could not find my carefully practiced technique! Slowly, oh so slowly, I pushed the needle in—aching with held breath, waiting for the shock of pain. It did not come. Certainly, while not having the professional hand of the nurses nor the mental toughness of my parents, I never have experienced the kind of pain I had feared. Sure, the shots have hurt on occasion over the years, but even my terrible technique of slowly pushing the needle in never has resulted in the pain I expected. Ah, what a relief!

The next anxiety attack I had over injections came when my parents announced that they were no longer going to assume primary responsibility for giving me my shots. During the week in the hospital, the nurses, my parents, and I had shared the responsibility. When we first returned home from Boston, Mom and Dad had been doing the dirty work. So I was not enthusiastic about their announcement. Oh, I knew the nurses had insisted that I be responsible for my own injections and had made my parents promise that they would not give me my shots, but I still didn't have much "confidence" in my own technique. I knew that it was my diabetes, but they were doing it "so well." I continued to protest. I guess they were not too crazy about my being clamped around their legs for the rest of their lives. My parents must have been listening when the nurses had encouraged them to not let me become dependent upon them for my diabetes care. I argued that making me give myself my shots cold turkey was cruel and unusual punishment. What difference did it make who gave the shots?

It wasn't like I had badgered them, but they did readily consent to buying me an automatic busher—a mechanical device that would give the injections.

The contraption arrived and the terror really set in. That spring-loaded device did not look like the lifesaver I thought it would be. It was about four inches of metal. The needle and syringe were inserted into the back of the device. The syringe rested on two guides on each side and was held in place by a rotating nut around the top near the plunger. The needle poked through two prongs at the end of the busher. To use the device, I had to lock in the syringe, cock the device by pulling it back against a spring, point the device by resting it on me (leg, stomach, thigh, or arm), and push the release. Wham, the needle seemed to fire into the leg.

"Well, ah, hmm. Do you think I might wait a while, ah . . . before I, ah, use that thing?" It looked lethal to me.

My parents held firm. I had to give myself the injections by hand or by the modern torture device. At first, I chose the hand— better that the agony be self-inflicted. That machine really did look cold, metallic, and lethal. But the pressure kept building as I slowly pushed the needle in each day and as the monster busher glared up from its box with the price tag still on it. I had these visions of the spring steel driving needle, syringe, and my father's Oldsmobile through my leg. But, despite my distaste for the machine and my real fears of its power, I was desperate for an alternative to my terribly slow hand.

I had to use it. My hand shook as I tightened down the depth guide for the third time. I bounced the syringe into the contraption. I cocked the spring. I set it all against my tender thigh. I waited and I waited and I waited. I could not bear to push the button. Finally, after what seemed like days, I gritted my teeth, closed my eyes, and pressed down the button. I did not hear myself scream. I did not hear my leg drop off. I did not hear the syringe twang into the floor. Not bad. I was going to use that sucker again. I retired Raymond's slow hand. Ah, what a relief!

All went well for about twelve years. My faithful busher and I had been through approximately 4,380 injections. We had become good friends; I depended upon it. As it turned out, I had become too dependent upon the contraption. One Sunday morning it broke. Bong! It was lifeless and useless. "Oh no!" I groaned. I knew that I would have to bring the slow hand out of retirement. I did not have the luxury of time to purchase a new busher, to work up my courage, or to brush up on my rusty technique. Plus we were fresh out of grapefruit. I had to have the shot then.

Although then nearly 23 years old, I still went through essentially the same experience that I had had in New England Deaconness Hospital. Where was the courage, the savior-faire, and the steely nerves that someone of my experience with diabetes ought to have? Hiding with my wife in the bedroom. Without the busher, the syringe felt as light as a feather. In fact, for some reason, it seemed to be waving in the air. It seemed so naked—it was naked! Yikes!

I waited and waited. The slow, hesitant pushing was all I had to offer my not-so-tender thigh. But I had to do it—and without the comfort of being able to close my eyes. To be sure though, I planned to grit my teeth. I wiped the spot a dozen times or so with the alcohol and cotton. I readied the syringe and waited. Time was flying. Oh well, slowly and gently I moved the needle into my skin and then the muscle. The insulin injected, I removed the needle quickly—almost the speed of light. Not bad. Ah, what a relief!

That was 22 years and approximately 17,790 shots ago, and I still go through periods of terror and fear about taking shots. First, because I wanted to avoid scarring and to enhance the absorption of my insulin, I decided to try out injection sites other than my thighs. I felt I needed to move around to my posterior, up to my stomach, and even occasionally into my skinny arms. Then there was the time I decided that I really should go to four injections a day. I wanted to watch and manage my glucose levels more carefully with the use of more frequent injections of Regular insulin. Once I was even in a situation where I had to use a bent needle. But, on each occasion, I have been able to sigh with relief.

Overall, I have not grown any fonder of needles and injections. I cannot even bear to see people on reruns of "M*A*S*H*" be given a shot. Nevertheless, from my experiences with injections and the recurring pattern of initial fear and then of relief, it has begun to occur to me that the worst part always has ended up being the awful anticipation. Never has an injection hurt as much as I had feared it would. Perhaps there is a lesson to be learned from all of this.

However, I must admit that after each of my four injections every day, I sigh and say, "Ah, what a relief!" I'm always glad it's over.

Food: Enemy or Ally?

For those of us with diabetes, food frequently presents a very real and a very troublesome conflict—we both love it and hate it.

On the one hand, food contains sugar and calories and therefore seems to be our enemy. Diet is a major ingredient in the treatment of diabetes. Doctors, nurses, nutritionists, family, and friends repeatedly hammer us with phrases such as "should you eat that," "don't eat such and such," "watch that diet," and "eat to live rather than live to eat." Each repetition focuses on food as the culprit. In contrast, every grocery store, television commercial, and magazine advertisement seems to feature "I'm-not-allowed-to-eat-that" items which torture even the most conscientious.

Meals are a hassle. A person who wrestles with counting calories or with food exchange lists for very long can turn downright surly. Counting or weighing or trying to tell what food goes into which group tests the patience of the saintly. Going into restaurants demands frantic searches through menus for selections that are not fried, not covered with mysterious sauces, or not so high in calories that a whole day's allotment is used up. Thus, whether at home or out, three-times-a-day meals serve to remind us that we have diabetes.

Food turns into reminders of restrictions, of inconveniences, and of an ominous future.

On the other hand, food can also seem an essential ally. First, food—for those with or without diabetes—is the source for physical nourishment. It contains the vital calories, vitamins, and minerals which provide fuel for running, growing, and healing the body. Food provides the complex combinations of protein, fat, and carbohydrates that sustain all people as they go to work or play, try to fight a cold or the flu, dare to think and create. Food seems the magic potion for a mysteriously effective organism. Without the essential nourishment, the marvelous body would starve and die. Food is health.

Second, food serves a crucial role in the functioning of most societies. Perhaps a sad commentary on contemporary life, meals provide a justification for families to get together. Whether it's the daily evening meal when father, mother, and the children have to abandon momentarily their individual schedules or a Thanksgiving feast when the whole clan gathers at someone's home to celebrate, food seems the central focus. Food is sharing.

Food and drink serve to oil the machinery of America's economy. Much of business is conducted at lunches, dinners, parties, and banquets where clients are entertained or employees are instructed or motivated. Many a deal is closed with a toast and canapes; many a program is launched over chicken and peas. Refreshments are served at company functions for the employees. Meals dominate America's corporate expense accounts. Food is one path to success.

Third, eating represents good times. People go out to eat to celebrate birthdays, anniversaries, promotions, and weekends. Coffee breaks—with accompanying snacks—give relief from a day's work or allow people to have some reason for sitting down and chatting with colleagues and friends. Vacations are occasions for culinary excess. From an early age, children eat their meals in order to get dessert. They are being "good" if they clean their plates. Cookies or cake or pie or candy turns into a tasty token of success. Win or lose, Little League games are followed by trips to Pizza Hut, Mr. Donut, or the snack bar. Television commercials bombard young and old with messages of "deserving a break today," enjoying the good life at elegant restaurants, and being a part of those-in-the-know who eat such and such a food at a designated fast food place. While frequently not healthy—full of empty calories, fat, and preservatives—food is fun.

Plus, food itself is a pleasant experience. It looks good sitting on the platter or in the dish. Its smells waft up to one's nose, triggering all sorts of sensory responses. Whether each item on the menu melts in the mouth or needs to be chewed, taste buds savor the temperatures, textures and flavors of each morsel. Each chew heightens every response. It can be heavenly! Food titillates the senses.

Food can also be symbolic. It represents to many people such things as security, love, or strength. Although not too many can still recall actually experiencing the depression which followed the 1929 stock market crash, the hardships associated with that era still hang over America. Images of the dust bowls, unemployment, poverty, and the resulting hunger haunt even those whose parents cannot remember the first manned space flight. Food can become a barrier used to protect us from those images and the fears associated with them. Parents, lovers, and friends give ice cream, candy, or fruit cake as expressions of love. The mere mention of Halloween, Valentine's Day, or Christmas evokes delicious images of wonderful experiences and food. Then, if one needs to get well or to get stronger, prescriptions include chicken soup or meat-and-potatoes. Food fills the stomach, suggests comfort, and builds the body. Food is security.

Indeed, people without diabetes may face the dilemma of food being both a threat to health as well a source of well-being. However, those of us with diabetes must face the seeming contradiction. We wrestle daily with food as an enemy and/or ally. With each meal or each injection or each exercise expedition or each doctor's visit, questions trouble us. What should we eat? How *much* should we eat? *When* should we eat? How will the food affect my blood sugar? These questions and many others rarely have simple, direct, or precise answers. Ambiguities and complexities provide little solace to those of us who are acutely aware of our own uncertain futures—especially when sugar levels are known to affect the length and quality of those futures.

In fact, we quickly discover that the very commodity that provides most other Americans with health, comfort, pleasure, and a sense of security represents the greatest threat to us. Even that concept isn't that simple: nourishment is essential; insulin reactions call for quick doses of simple sugars; certain foods are "free"; others reduce insulin requirements; particular combinations in increased qualities should be eaten before exercise.

Just working out the biological formula has baffled experts for years. To add in the fact that those with diabetes are also people with the emotional and psychological needs like the rest of America makes the dilemmas of food unbelievably complex. We also want and need the emotional nourishing that comes with food in America. We want to feel strong, to feel safe, to savor the sensations, and to participate in the social rituals associated with food.

Why can't we enjoy the freedom, the desserts, the restaurants, and the sense of fitting in with the crowd?

Somehow reducing food to "don't eat that," "you're allowed only this much of that," or "stick to 1600 calories" isn't even somewhat adequate. Life and food are not that simple for anyone. As a person with diabetes, I find food befuddling and frustrating. I love food and I hate food—frequently at the same time.

Eating with the Ignorant, the Insensitive, and the Well-Meaning

I STILL CAN REMEMBER WHEN, as a youngster in the fourth grade, I returned to school two weeks after being diagnosed as having diabetes. A class party happened to be going on that morning. Mothers spread out the goodies as my classmates put finishing touches on the decorations. As the festivities geared up to a dull roar, a classmate who knew I had diabetes tip-toed up to me at my desk. He timidly extended his right hand. "Can you eat this?" he whispered. His tiny hand held a pathetically small piece of chewing gum.

That experience was the first of a long line that I call "eating with the ignorant, the insensitive, and the well-meaning." People are forever trying to help me with my diet. Usually these efforts result in my discomfort and embarrassment. On occasion, the "help" pushes me to deny my diabetes and to ignore my diet.

The ignorant, the insensitive, and the well-meaning know that diabetes has something to do with food. So it seems that every time we have a meal together, go for a coffee break, meet at a party, or drive by a grocery store, the unsolicited help comes. Most frequently the help comes as a battery of questions.

"Can you eat this?"

"Is this on your diet?"

"How much of this can you eat?"

"Can you drink?"

"What can you drink?"

"How many calories are you allowed on your diet?"

"Are you sure that this fits into your diet? Don't you think that it has too many calories? Should you be eating this?"

"Where should we go to eat? Is there a place that has the food you can eat?"

"Do you mind if I order dessert?"

"Isn't it awful that you can't eat what you want?"

"Do you know that I feel very guilty about eating this in front of you?"

"Have you tried any of those special dietetic or diabetic foods? Don't they make it easier for you?"

"Can't you just take more insulin?"

How does one answer such questions in 25 words or less? How does one respond politely and without hostility? Who wants to detail the entire process of metabolism? Does every meal have to be a short course in diabetes? If you answer one question, that always seems to lead to another and another. Even one of these questions is enough to make me self-conscious while I am trying to eat. Who wouldn't feel as if the rest of the world were focusing upon his every bite? It's tough enjoying a meal.

Help sometimes comes in the form of special preparations. On occasion when I have been invited to a party or out for a meal, the host or hostess will have gone out of his or her way to prepare something special for me and my diabetes. I can recall on one occasion when my plate held only rabbit food: not one calorie could be found among the greens, the yellows, and the blands. Then there was a meal totally void of carbohydrates, only meats and cheeses. At a dinner honoring a retiring colleague attended by the rest of the department and their spouses, I was the only one to get an appetizer— a grapefruit. The hostess had heard somewhere that "diabetics have to eat grapefruit before every meal." The amount of dietary misinformation floating around about diabetes is astounding. Unfortunately, it seems to me that I am the primary victim of most of it.

More embarrassing are the announcements which usually come with the "special food for the diabetic." "Oh Mike," in a whisper that can be heard across the street, "don't worry, you won't have to eat the delicious roast beef and stuffed potatoes. I've made a *diabetic* salad just for you." Or "We are all having brandy and chocolate mousse. May I get you a small apple?" Sometimes I just cringe. Other times, out of spite, I have eaten three portions of the "normal people's food." Once—during one of my more mature evenings—I did not eat a thing.

I know—not very intelligent.

I know that the vast majority of people are ignorant of the intricacies involved with managing a diet that helps keep the sugar levels down and sustains the body's functions for someone with diabetes.

I know that many people are insensitive to the implications of what they say to or do for people with diabetes. Not having the disease, they do not consider what they do or say. It does not occur to them that it might hurt the feelings of those with diabetes, that it might make them feel uncomfortable, or that it could trip some internal mechanism which incites rebellion or denial.

I know that most people are well-meaning in their endeavors to help. Their special efforts to provide "safe" food are genuine; their questions are honest; their sympathy is sincere. How could they be aware of the possible effects their efforts might have on someone with diabetes?

I know about the hazards of eating with the ignorant, the insensitive, and the well-meaning. I may even know why it is so hazardous.

I know that—having recognized the hazards—a mature person would try to develop strategies for dealing with these people.

I have tried to limit the emotional carnage. With the ignorant, I tell myself that they don't know any better. In fact, a great many people know very little about nutrition and many other things related to diabetes. Why should they be expected to? How much do I know about cars, adoption, or even narcolepsy? With the insensitive, I remind myself that I tend to be thin-skinned about language in general and diabetes in particular. As the questions pour forth, I mutter to myself, "Lighten up, lighten up." Why read so much into what they do or say? What they ask or say isn't meant to be an affront to my manhood, gene pool, or personal worth. The well-meaning—I know—are caring people acting out of kindness. My strategy with them is to use the "gift cliché"—it's the thought that counts. Like some of the ties I've received, their help may be ugly and out of style, but their intentions are good.

I also have developed strategies for preventing catastrophes to my glucose levels. Asking what sort of get-together is planned can help: frequently the host or hostess will divulge if it is to be a meal or snacks and even what type of food is to be served. I usually wait until arriving where I am to eat and discovering what is to be offered before taking my injection. Sometimes, when I know what the bill of fare is to be, I take my shot and eat something at home beforehand. At the host's meal, I nibble at what will complete an appropriate meal for me and my health. I also have taken to heart the recent trends in assertiveness training by merely declining to eat without explanation what is not good for me. The diabetes need not be mentioned; therefore the awkward questions can be avoided. Furthermore, lots of people are health-conscious and/or are on diets these days. As a result, those giving a party are less likely to be offended by questions concerning ingredients or by a guest's decision not to partake of some dish. Another strategy is to bring a snack with me just in case the meal offered doesn't provide what I need.

But, despite these strategies, I still can't help but cringe when I know that I will be eating with the ignorant, the insensitive, and the well-meaning.

Read Those Labels

For MANY YEARS, I have been going to a local restaurant for lunch. The food is rather ordinary, but the people are friendly. Plus going out to lunch provides an opportunity to get away from work for a peaceful hour.

One day I couldn't get anyone to go to lunch with me, and I neglected to bring along something to read. So, while I awaited my chef's salad and sipped my iced tea, I began reading the empty pink packet of artificial sweetener that I had dumped into the tea.

I could not believe what I was reading. First of all, it contained 3.5 calories. That did not seem like a lot, but it certainly was more than I had thought it would contain.

The shock, however, was the amount of carbohydrates: 8.7 grams. Eight-point-seven grams of carbohydrates crammed into a single little pink packet of supposed "sugar substitute"! I had been drinking three, four, or five glasses of iced tea with every lunch. That can be as many as 43.5 grams of carbohydrates. A hamburger at Burger King has only 23 grams of carbohydrates; a Big Mac at MacDonald's contains 44 grams; a whole Rancher platter at Burger Chef provides 44 grams. To get the carbohydrates of three packets of the advertised artificial sweetener, I could eat a tostada or two tacos at Taco Bell.

While the pink packet certainly did not contain the grams of protein and of fat in the notorious fast foods nor the calories, the point is that I had assumed that the artificial sweetener was essentially nutritionally free. For years and years, meal after meal, I had been pouring the stuff into too many glasses of iced tea and too many cups of coffee. (Caffeine is my one dietary sin.)

I had not taken the time to investigate. I had just used it without bothering to see what it was. Because this particular brand is packaged like the other brands with its small pink packet and its "sugar substitute" label, I assumed it was like the rest. I ignored the tiny little numbers printed on each and every packet I had ripped open and poured into my drinks.

If I am going to consume so many grams of carbohydrates, I want to know that I am doing it. There is nothing like trying to balance diet, insulin, and exercise and having uncounted carbohydrates sneaking into the equation. Furthermore, if amounts of my daily allotment of carbohydrates are to be used up, I don't want them being wasted on packets of artificial sweeteners that leave an aftertaste. Too many foods with the same amount of carbohydrates exist that taste much, much better.

The lesson for me is that those of us with diabetes should be more careful about the assumptions we make about packaged food. I need to continue to pay attention no matter how much experience I have had with assorted food products.

Eating is too much fun and too important to me to be done carelessly. I do not want food to become the enemy in my treatment of my diabetes. Handling the disease is difficult enough without allowing one part of it to become an adversary. Sneak attacks in surprising little pink packets are experiences that tend to make me very suspicious of food. How long have they been sabotaging my efforts for control?

From now on, I will be carrying packets of artificial sweeteners that are not hidden carbohydrates. I also will be reading food labels.

Those Damned Machines!

For years I have been at best uncomfortable with machines of any sort. The discomfort is so great that I still have the same two cars I have ever bought. It isn't because I love the old models; they frequently don't run. It's just that I don't want to have to learn the quirks of new machines. My VW Bug and Rabbit limp along without any hopes for retirement because I just can't face the challenges of a new machine in my life.

Therefore, my response to such suggestions as buying a mechanical device for monitoring my blood sugars or going onto an insulin pump to better control my sugars has not surprised anyone who knows me at all.

"No way! Never!"

Many reasons (rationalizations?) occasioned such a refusal to consider either device. First of all, I am cheap—as in tightfisted, stingy, or miserly. Today's machines cost big bucks—from hundreds to thousands of dollars—and I was reluctant to part with that kind of money. Too many times I have seen acquaintances rush out to buy the latest mechanical invention to trim their hedges, produce memorable movies of the family, or allow them to communicate with the entire trucking industry and have the expensive trinkets serve only to hang around and remind them that not all Americans are mechanical engineers. The money seemed better spent on luxury items like food, clothing, gasoline, mortgages, and the amenities associated with having diabetes.

Second, I had never found machines very friendly. "User-friendly" isn't a part of my vocabulary. Machines and I have always had an adversarial relationship: they didn't like me, so I hated them. More often than not, my cars won't start, the bank's computers seem more often to be "down" than working, and my television goes on the blink just before the big game. Furthermore, when the car radio conks out or the lawn mower won't even sputter, the machines can't or won't communicate with me. They won't tell me what is wrong with them when they don't (or won't) work. They are so cold, so mechanical, and so detached. They don't seem the least bit concerned that they are ruining my day.

Machines always seemed to work on some mysterious principle that they insist on keeping to themselves. No matter how carefully I read the directions, listened to the repeated demonstrations, and tried to do it correctly, I couldn't develop any confidence when using a machine. I could not get any of them to work as promised. I could almost hear them chuckling at me.

Third, I was reluctant to surrender any of my life to the dictates of a machine. To me, life is meant to be, among other things, spontaneous and flexible. Tight scheduling, rigid procedures, statistical data, and mechanical parts hardly seem to infuse life with vitality. As a person more comfortable with books and people than with science and numbers, I had trouble seeing myself integrating a monitor or a pump into my life. Perhaps I am old-fashioned: I had preferred to snuggle up with another human being than with a microprocessor. It seemed unnatural to have a machine tell me what to do. How could I have a machine attached to me throughout each day? What if I finally came up with something wild or exciting to do? What would I do with a glucose monitor or an insulin pump?

Not me—no machines. I'd have bet the ranch that I would never subject myself to such machines.

So much for "never." There goes the ranch.

I took the plunge and bought a battery-operated blood glucose monitor. While many models exist (with a variety of accessories, sizes, capabilities, costs, and testing procedures), mine is small (5½" x 2¾" x ⅛") and light (about 4.5 ounces without the six-volt battery). It cost $109 without rebate or trade-in: that included the monitor, a battery, a bottle of test strips, a lancet device, a carrying case, a user's manual, a VCR instruction tape, a pocket-sized testing guide, and a self-test diary for recording results.

After inserting the calibration strip from the bottle of test strips (only necessary with each new bottle of strips), I have discovered the testing pretty simple—even for me. All I have to do is turn on the machine, prick my finger with the lancet device, place a drop of blood on a test strip, touch the timing button, wait 60 seconds, wipe the blood off the strip, put the strip in the machine, and wait another 60 seconds. Presto! The machine gives me my blood glucose level. My monitor seems made for me—it "beeps" every time something has to be done, it tells me on its display if something has gone awry, and it tells me the day and time when I am using it. Clearly a machine for an absent-minded machine-hater!

Before I reveal how I—the great machine-hater—came to be converted, I must confess that I am delighted with the device. The blood glucose monitor has turned out to be worth the cost and the time to learn how to use it because it is positively liberating.

It has reduced the stress I feel while striving to manage my diabetes because it provides specific numerical sugar readings. I no longer have to twist and turn in front of a variety of lights trying to read frequently ambiguous shades of color on test strips for visual testing. Gone are such eternal questions of "is it closer to 180 or 240?" and "how much over 240 is it?" The 400-to-800 range would test the keenest eyesight. What does a 450 look like? a 500? a 700? With the machine, the guesswork is gone and the insulin scales have been refined to be adapted to specific shifts in sugar levels.

Checking the sugar is less arduous with the machine: I am more willing to do it. With the visual method, I had to put the blood on the strip, scramble for my watch, stare at the second hand for a full minute, wipe the blood off the strip, wait another minute, compare the colors on the strip with the chart on the strips' container, and then begin the guessing. With the machine—including beeps, timer, and messages—monitoring is easier. So is managing the diabetes. Controlling the sugars has become a more exact science: I find that I am less easily discouraged while seeking the elusive control.

Furthermore, by relinquishing most of the testing task to the machine, I have permitted myself the silly—but effective—delusion that whatever the test results it's the machine's fault. Sure, I know that it is my excessive eating, my lack of exercise, or my having given myself too much insulin which makes the numbers too high or too low. But I find it easier for me to say "that damn machine" or "machines are idiots" than to start abusing myself. With the machine as a silly scapegoat upon which to heap the abuse, I am freed to take the data and to approach the glucose level with a more detached, problem-solving approach. By yelling at a machine that has no feelings to be hurt, I can unload my anger, disappointment, or frustration without ending up sulking or pouting. I "clear the air" and move on try to meet the challenge. It is not very realistic, but the delusion allows me to respond to the numbers less emotionally.

However, the significance of this story does not rest primarily in the amazing turnaround in my attitude toward the machine nor in the freedom gained from using a machine that I had strongly resisted. A greater significance comes from how I arrived at the conversion and the resulting sense of freedom.

Four people in their own ways contributed to the turnaround.

First, there was Beth, a diabetes nurse specialist. She gently but persistently urged me to consider the value of using the machine for increased control. By using the monitor, she explained, I would have a fairly accurate knowledge of my blood glucose levels before meals and bedtime or whenever I tested myself. That way I could evaluate my insulin doses, my diet, my exercise routines, and my levels of stress in light of my "sugars" and then make adjustments based on the monitor's readings. Not only could I control my glucose levels more carefully, but I also would have a sense of being in control.

Beth never pushed: she encouraged me to voice as strongly as I wanted my objections to machines. She never ridiculed what must have seemed to her to be immature or emotional rationalizations. She even refused to argue with me about how irrational my opposition was. She was patient. For over a year, she used the machine in my presence and indirectly suggested the possible benefits others had enjoyed from using the monitor. She even went out of her way to make an acquisition—if I decided to do it—seem easy. Beth set the stage by providing the information about the machine and the reasons for using it without making it all into a life-or-death campaign. As I resisted month after month the very mention of machines, Beth allowed me to discover for myself the possibilities a monitor might have and waited for me to decide if I might consider giving it a try. Clearly, if I were to take the plunge, it would be my choice.

Next, there was Maggie, a delightful person with diabetes who had managed to go through the wars and had retained her sense of humor and zest for life. Time and again, Maggie and I shared our distaste for machines such as the glucose monitor. Right in the middle of a diabetes care unit where the nurses used them day in and day out, we joked and made snide remarks about "those damned machines." We would catalog our objections almost as a ritual during each get-together: the machines were expensive, cumbersome, mechanical, inhibiting, etc., etc., etc. Maggie and I were kindred spirits, and the machine-resistance had been just another instance of our ties.

Fortunately, Maggie did not remain as stubborn as I. One day I wandered into the unit to discover her trying out a monitor that used half of one test strip. Much to my surprise, she had been experimenting with the machine for several days and had not been able to break it.

"Not too bad," she admitted. "You know, I am not finding this to be as much as an ordeal as I thought it would be. I don't exactly love it, but I may give it a chance."

"Not me," I announced. I then listed my well-worn objections and made some reference to hell freezing over before I would buy "one of those things."

"Yeah, I know. I'm not sure, but I am willing to give it a shot."

"Okay," I laughed.

But Maggie's experiment started me to think about reevaluating my position. We had shared too much about how it is to have diabetes to just dismiss her willingness to give it a try. I had admired her as a person ever since I had known her. I knew that her outlook on life was much like mine—if not stronger about refusing to surrender any part of her life to others or to machines. I found myself thinking about it more and more.

The next time I saw her we discussed her further experiences with "it." She did not paint her experiences as spiritual experiences, but did indicate that she was still willing to "see how it goes." I told her that, if she actually got one, I might consider trying out a glucose monitor. She restrained herself from falling over in shock.

Then a little medical adventure required that I spend some time in the hospital. During my stay, Beth provided the health care (which included the use of the monitor), and Maggie came armed with her extraordinary support.

Before I knew it, I had agreed to give the glucose monitor a chance. This brought the third person's crucial contribution to my turnaround. Mary, a perky diabetes teaching nurse specialist, allowed me to learn how to use the machine with comfort. Having known Mary from a previous stay in the hospital, I was comfortable with her, but, when she bounced into my room, I had no sense of an "upcoming lesson" or confrontation with a machine.

Mary didn't merely hand me the machine and the user's manual. She ran through the procedure herself, giving "insider's" pointers as she went along. Any step which might seem tricky was explained in terms of how she had learned from her own experiences. She provided ample opportunities for questions or paused when I seemed just a little puzzled.

Then she turned the machine over to me to give it a try. Since it wasn't time for a scheduled glucose check to determine my next insulin dosage, I felt less pressure. I could concentrate just on learning how to use the new machine. Step-by-step, we went through the procedure that she had demonstrated to me. Anxious and hesitant about using the machine, I fumbled through the procedure. Mary did not intervene, criticize, or even raise her eyebrows. As I staggered through each unfamiliar step, she encouraged me with wide smiles and comments such as "that's it," "good work," or "you've got it." When I did make an error, an "I've done that myself a number of times" quickly reassured me.

Mary continued her upbeat, positive approach as she induced me to repeat several practice sessions with the new machine. Each run-through was more and more successful; with increasing ease and efficiency, I grew more and more comfortable with one of those "damned machines."

"Great. You're a natural. A quick study."

Mary beamed. I smiled in appreciation of an educator who focused on a "pupil's" learning rather than on her teaching.

The fourth individual's contribution to the conversion came later—as a result of Beth's, Maggie's, and Mary's help—but it was vital. It was mine.

No matter how much information, how much encouragement, how much support, and how much education a person receives, none of it is very valuable unless the person who is the object of it all is receptive and willing to give it a try. New treatments— whether with a new machine, a new insulin, a new diet, or a new drug—can seem unsettling if not threatening. No amount of careful reasoning, research data, loving support, or refined teaching is enough to overcome patient resistance. Although each can contribute to bringing a person to the brink of change, he or she must make that last small step and take a risk.

Ultimately, I decided to give that "damned machine" a try.

Nourished and encouraged by Beth, Maggie, and Mary, my decision gave me a chance to feel that I was able to gain better control while feeling freer, even though I am still doing the glucose monitoring. But there would not have been that chance without my willingness finally to be receptive to Beth, Maggie, and Mary.

Who knows, perhaps as a team, the four of us might work together on my considering another one of "those damned machines"—an insulin pump?

The Usual Unreliable Sources

Reading the newspaper can be hazardous to one's health.

Not too long ago, a heartwarming wire service story appeared in the local newspaper. The story told of a girl who had won something like $75,000 and had donated all or part of it to the Juvenile Diabetes Foundation for research. The story went on to tell how the girl herself had juvenile diabetes and how one with such a disease could not expect to live through her twenties.

Upon reading this story, I nearly keeled over into a death rattle. I have had diabetes since I was nine and was now in my mid-forties. According to the news story, I should have been dead for about two decades!

Another soul-twisting news story focused on a kidney transplant operation for a pretty young girl. The story told of a long-absent father coming forward to provide the vital organ and to save the girl from renal failure and daily dialysis. The father had divorced the girl's mother more than a decade before, had moved out of the country, and had not been heard from for many years. In her time of need, however, he returned to assist the teenager, who also was blind. With accompanying photographs, the story delivered the punch line that her physical conditions were due to diabetes.

Having insulin-dependent diabetes, I could only cringe, blink my eyes, and grieve for my kidneys.

Even newspaper stories that describe the successes of people with diabetes can send us and our families into despair and anxieties about life-threatening symptoms. For example, a local elementary school student who happened to have diabetes had just been selected to attend a governor's conference for gifted students in the state capital. In the story describing the young scholar's abilities and activities, her diabetes received considerable attention. As if showing how the student's assets are balanced off by the deficits of having the disease, the story painted the "sad prospects of having diabetes."

Such paragraphs could mar anyone's pleasure in the victories of life; for a person with diabetes, they ensure the recollection of the grim details of living with the disease.

Such are the hazards of reading the newspaper. Journalism is a peculiar profession in that, while usually committed to the truth, it is restricted by the amount of space it can give a story, by the shape that the story can take, by the need to sell newspapers, and by the level of expertise a reporter can have concerning subjects such as medicine. As a result of these restrictions, stories such as those mentioned above can be inaccurate, distort the facts, or leave the readers with improper impressions.

Even if they are accurate, clear, and dependable, newspaper stories on diabetes can stir a variety of responses from us with the disease. The responses may range from mere despair to full terror. Some have reported developing symptoms described in certain stories. Others have had positive, aggressive approaches to their diabetes undercut by stories reminding them of complications and disasters tied to diabetes.

The power of the press can be devastating. We should be very careful not to succumb too readily to such power. Unchecked by those most effected, the power of misinformation, half truths, and incomplete data can upset the delicate balance necessary for handling diabetes and for living with the disease. Anyone who has had any experience with having diabetes—or treating those who do— knows that the emotional or psychological side of the disease is as crucial as the hardcore medical side.

But journalism isn't the only culprit that can upset the delicate balance. How many times have we been told of such-and-such a person with diabetes who did everything wrong—ate chocolate cake for three meals a day, drank a quart of scotch regularly, never adjusted the insulin, and exercised only when running away from doctors—and lived to be eighty-five-years old without a single complication? Then there is the other story, the one who did it all by the book—followed the diet, monitored the glucose levels, adjusted the insulin, exercised everyday, and did whatever the doctor recommended—and suffered every complication in the book (and some yet undiscovered) and died in the prime of youth.

Such accounts can send us into tailspins just as easily as do inaccurate or insensitive newspaper stories. Stories reporting extreme cases can be damaging because they make it sound like moderation does not exist. They imply that therapeutic systems don't work and that treating diabetes is a game of chance. "Why bother?" we ask, "when control really doesn't matter?" When considered rationally, it doesn't make sense to respond to such extreme unreliable stories, but we do. I have—hook, line, and sinker—many, many times.

Even stories that avoid the worst scenario and the best scenario can produce undesirable results. True stories can be almost as unreliable. Sometimes, while telling their own stories or trying to give support to another with diabetes, people can get carried away with the graphic details of their particular ordeals. The details may include accounts of operations, pains, setbacks, and bizarre occurrences connected with diabetes. Sometimes the details are absolutely accurate; other times the storytellers might dramatize their narrative. Whether completely true or not, they can adversely affect two groups the audience and the storyteller.

Upon hearing the story, an unsuspecting audience can select details from the reported ordeal and apply them to themselves. Frequently, the application of the details is totally inappropriate: the medical histories may differ; the life styles may not be the same; other circumstances may have been left out. But we launch into a full-scale adoption of the entire story. Many times such conversations have left me aching, limping, and suffering with symptoms that didn't exist prior to the conversation. Even if the physical symptoms are not assumed, the worries about having them can create all sorts of problems. A mere headache can be turned into a stroke, sore muscles into neuropathy, indigestion into a heart attack, an infected insect bite into a potential amputation. Accounts of insulin reactions can result in overeating and high sugars for weeks as the audience tries to avoid repeating the reported experiences. Who would exercise after someone has told how he fell on his face from low sugar while just walking? There are enough problems managing our own diabetes without taking on the problems related by someone else.

The storytellers themselves can suffer from their own stories. As they go back over some unfortunate incident—whether open-heart surgery or the removal of an ingrown toenail, a severe insulin reaction or a high sugar for no apparent reason—they also are re-experiencing the gamut of emotions. They can relive the fears, the discomfort, the embarrassment, and the disappointments that came with the experiences. The reliving of the experiences and their emotional impact, in turn, can intimidate the storytellers. In light of the experiences recalled, why risk the associated traumas? Who would venture again into life's mainstream if certain mishaps are so common? The retelling of the problems can embed them into the tellers' consciousness of diabetes and can inhibit their willingness to try things again or to live fully.

Thus, in many ways, most unsolicited information about diabetes and living with diabetes can be hazardous to those who accept it without reservation. Sometimes the information is inaccurate or incomplete. Even if the information is correct, its impact may have adverse effects as it lets loose untapped emotional monsters.

To avoid such pitfalls, I try to remind myself that the newspaper or the storyteller may be wrong. Sources are not always reliable. I insist on checking out the information through other sources such as doctors, nurses, or articles in medical journals before getting upset. Knowing what is accurate or that I have all the information available helps me adjust or respond to new input into my diabetes management.

If the data turns out to be accurate, I still try not to accept it as the gospel for myself. Listeners are not always reliable. I strive to prevent my usual emotional overreaction to news about diabetes. I tell myself that just because someone else or a group of people had such experiences does not insure that I too must go through it. Even if I know for certain that such-and-such an experience is going to happen to me, I tell myself that there is no point getting into an uproar about something there is nothing I can do. Why compound a problem with rage, stress, or other uncontrolled responses?

Of course, these steps are what I try to do when confronted with stories associated with diabetes. I am not always successful. All too often I go off the deep end when I chance upon stories without warning.

I am still working on remembering that on most occasions these stories come from the "usual unreliable sources."

Hemoglobin A1C: Punishing Test or Magic Gateway?

I USUALLY SKIP DOWN to the mailbox. Under normal circumstances, I view that silver box as a magic gateway to the outside world. It brings messages from distant friends, creative strategies to get me to spend my money, persistent efforts to collect after I have succumbed to the strategies, and a cornucopia of magazines and journals.

But, at one time, the journey wasn't under normal circumstances. A few days earlier I had gone for a long overdue regular three-month checkup. For some stranger reason—actually I was too chicken to object—I had submitted to the usual blood drawing. I knew what they wanted with that test tube of my precious blood: a blood sugar and a hemoglobin A1C. The blood sugar report would be immediate; the HA1C would come in the mail.

The hemoglobin A1C is a test that measures a person's control over his or her blood glucose for an extended period of time. Specifically, it measures how much sugar (glucose) attaches to hemoglobin, an element in the blood. It seems that the glucose sticks to the hemoglobin and therefore allows the measurement of sugar levels over a span of time. Unlike the blood sugar test, the HA1C cannot be manipulated for special occasions by temporary starvation, excessive exercise, and massive insulin dosages. It provides a broad view of a diabetes treatment program by indicating overall effectiveness levels rather than one sugar level at one point in time. The results are reported in percentages. Usually the percentages are grouped in ranges that reflect the quality of glucose control over the previous two to three months. For example, my doctor considers 10-18% as "poor" control, 9-10% "fair," 7. 5-9% "good," and 2-7. 5% "excellent."

Even at that, the HA1C does not stand alone as the "be-all-and-end-all" measure of the effectiveness of diabetes control. Many times I have been told that I also should consider a number of other factors: How do I feel emotionally and physically? How is my weight? Am I too thin or too fat? Have there been any major changes recently? The home glucose monitoring should not be ignored. If I have been checking the sugars four times a day for four to six days a week, those numbers should provide a reliable indication of my control.

While in the doctor's office, I was certain the results of the blood sugar and the HA1C would be disastrous. I wasn't wrong about the blood sugar: despite my 150 at noon, a boosted insulin dosage, and a moderate lunch, it read a cranky 235. That number really wasn't too bad considering what my blood glucose monitor had been screaming at me lately. From my perception, I could count on one hand the number of times my "sugars" had been in the 80-120 mg/dl "normal" range—and have several fingers left over.

"God," I thought. "No telling what the HA1C will be. Thank goodness I'll be long gone by the time they get that result."

That prayer of thanks, of course, had not taken into consideration that I would get the results in due time. That's why the mailbox had lost its appeal. It no longer seemed to be the magic gateway. Any day it would bring the HA1C results. Certainly, the doctor and the nurses wouldn't be there to give me hell, but I still was afraid.

I was certain that my latest HA1C would document a somewhat-less-than-ideal implementation of my diabetes management program. For various reasons—eating binges, insulin reactions, increased stress at work, an infection, tennis tournaments, a couple of beers at poker—my blood sugars had been going up and down like a yo-yo: 400+ to 60 to 400+. I just knew that, when I opened the mailbox with the doctor's little report, it would roar out, "You jerk! You have been pigging out at Mr. Donut, sitting around on your biggest part watching television, and generally ignoring all of our advice!" I wouldn't have been surprised if a guy in a white medical coat and 98-inch shoulders were to leap out of the mailbox and start lashing me. Perhaps we could move or I could merely remove the mailbox itself, or we could take a long vacation in the Amazon jungle.

But, before I could decide which protective measure to take, our surly mailperson rolled up to #2422 and deposited the feared report. Was the box rumbling? Was that the earth shaking? Could I hear muffled roars? I inched my way down the path. I held the box's handle, worked up my courage, decided to take my medicine like a grown-up, and pulled down. There it was, glowering among the postcard from Grandma Phyllis, the Sears bill, the 436th offer of a free camera if I would look at a great condominium, and *Newsweek*. I read everything before I touched the report. Twice.

Silly me! The cute little scale and the written report indicated an 8%—seemingly just between excellent control and good control. Whew! I howled in delight. The family rushed out of the house with anxious looks on their faces. "Let's go out to lunch!" I announced. After the enthusiasm waned, I wondered about my response to the latest encounter with the HA1C and my history with the test. For over three years I had been "taking the test."

When I first came out of the closet with my diabetes, my first HA1C was done in the hospital. It was almost in triple digits. I suffered with severe guilt because of my criminal life of denial, ice-cold Cokes, strawberry cheesecake, and marbled roast beef. I felt like my mug was on posters in all the post offices in America. I had been bad, and I had been caught. Everyone knew what a criminal I was and had been. I could just see their sneers of contempt. I was marked for a premature death and for terminal stupidity.

The second HA1C was taken about six months after I had launched myself upon a vigorous reclamation project. With the teachings and help of several diabetes educators and my friends, I had committed myself to a diabetes management program. This test would document our progress. Before the test, I was very nervous: Had the efforts been worth it? Would I let down all who had helped so much? Would there be progress and therefore hope? If the results were good, would the sneers disappear? If they were bad, would everyone assume that I had been cheating or that I had not really been working hard on managing my diabetes? After the test, I was disappointed. Although no longer in triple digits and certainly in the high-normal range, the results did not reflect—in my estimation—the amount of work that I had put into turning things around. What more could I do? Was I destined for disaster?

Another experience I have had with the HA1C is the non-experience. During a routine visit to the doctor, I declined to have any blood drawn. I had done a glucose self-monitoring at lunch and my appointment was at 1:00 P.M. Why do another one so soon? I also resisted the request for a HA1C. I felt that I had been keeping careful track of my blood sugars with home self-monitoring four times a day and with a detailed record of the sugars, the insulin dosages, the exercise, and other influencing factors. I knew how things were going—I didn't need another test. This non-experience—I suspect—resulted from more than my rational explanations. Beyond the economic savings and the avoidance of repeating data collection, my "reasons" probably also developed from an unconscious mixture of the responses experienced the first two times with the HA1C. Perhaps I wanted some time off from the guilt, the sneers, and the disappointment. I was avoiding documentation that I had been screwing up or that the results could always be better.

In my mind, no ambiguity existed with the latest HA1C: I did not want to face the test and its results. I didn't want the hard evidence for my guilt. Nor did I want the recriminations of others on top of my own. I didn't want the "tutt-tutt," the "that's too bad," the "we should try harder," or the "you know that control decreases the chances for complications with diabetes."

But what I got was a surprise. The catastrophic results were not there. Nor was the guilt, the fear, or the disappointment. Clearly, my perception of my diabetes management had been selective. I had remembered only the slips and the high glucose readings; I had not kept the "big picture" in view. I had been too hard on myself, too insistent on perfection. As the HA1C documented, I had been doing better than I had thought.

With the surprise came an entirely new vision of the HA1C. "Hey, I'm not doing too badly! Way to go, Raymond! That HA1C isn't so bad after all! Boy, I know I can do better because the control hasn't been that good. Wait until the next HA1C—I'll knock the socks off of it!"

How quickly one forgets. Despair to hope in a flash. Clearly for me, the HA1C assumes many emotional identities—depending upon the results. I think this is because, when it boils down, I see the HA1C test as just that—a test. It is a lie detector, a report card, a way of checking up. It is a threat to my well-being, an enemy.

Another surprise. As an English teacher, I tell my students that tests are opportunities. On tests, they can show what they have learned. They can discover what they do not know and therefore have a chance to correct the oversight. They can see the process of taking tests as a way of applying what they have learned and therefore discovering new things that aren't memorized. They can gain confidence in what they do know, in how they perform under pressure, and in how they measure up to societal demands. As an English teacher, I tell my students that a test should be seen as a tool for dealing with the future more than a record of the past. Because they have had an unfortunate experience on a particular test, they should not despair. There will be more tests: one test does not mean the end of the world. One test does not condemn them to a life of failure or even mediocrity. It can provide a guideline for future preparations—how to study, what to study, what field is not one of their strengths. Tests should be seen as an open-ended opportunity for growth rather than as an instrument for punishment.

Perhaps I need to examine the discrepancy between how I see tests in my classroom and how I see the HA1C. Perhaps the HA1C provides as many opportunities as I hope my tests do. Perhaps the HA1C need not be synonymous with fear, guilt, disappointment, and despair. Could it also be a tool for dealing with the future?

Could my mailbox always be a magic gateway?

Watch Your Language!

AT A RECENT DIABETES support group meeting, a man about my age described how he felt about his diabetes.

"I don't mind being a DIABETIC. I lead a fairly NORMAL life. . . . I have adjusted pretty well to not being NORMAL. . . . I try to do as many NORMAL activities as possible. . . . If we are very careful and keep tight control, we may lead fairly NORMAL lives."

As he continued talking, I was developing a dislike for a man I barely knew. Later, it occurred to me what had gotten under my skin. I didn't like the language he used. Oh, he didn't offend the English teacher in me: his grammar and usage were flawless.

I didn't like his word choice.

I took exception to his use of the word NORMAL. What does NORMAL mean? Doesn't his use of the word NORMAL imply that people with diabetes are ABNORMAL. The word NORMAL suggested to me that people with diabetes are have-nots or outsiders or inferior. Clearly, to me, the word NORMAL seemed stupid, harsh, insensitive, and cruel.

People with or without diabetes, it seems to me, should consider the impact of their use of the word "normal." In fact, anyone dealing with people in general as well as with those with diabetes should reflect on the use of "normal."

When doctors, diabetes educators, family members, friends, and people with diabetes use the word "normal," they thrust people with diabetes into a world apart. They signal that "diabetics" are "different." They imply that a life with diabetes is totally unlike the one that everyone else enjoys. The word "normal" sends contrasting images through the mind: a life without cares and a life of diets, shots, and fear; one of freedom and one of restrictions; one of perfection and happiness, and one of imperfection and despair.

Those carelessly using the word "normal" also create a vision of an unattainable goal. What is "normal"? Who is "normal"? Who is to say what is "normal"? Does "normal" exist? Without specific answers, people who are told directly or indirectly that they aren't "normal" are left to imagine what it is that they do not have. Thus the state of being "normal" takes on gigantic mystical proportions for those who aren't. They focus on what they aren't rather than what they are. They ache to be "normal."

The word "normal" can create problems more serious than disappointed dreams. It can obstruct effective treatment of diabetes. People don't want to be abnormal. To imply that having diabetes keeps them from being "normal" can ensure denial of the very existence of the disease. It is tough treating a disease when we will not admit having it. Furthermore, coupling "normal" with the objectives in controlling diabetes—such as "normal blood sugars" or "normal activities"—can contribute to noncompliance. People aching to be "normal," happy, and carefree tend to avoid anything which reminds them that they are different. Testing a blood sugar provides the opportunity of revealing an abnormally high sugar and therefore a reminder that they have diabetes and are different and apart—so why test? Telling them that noncompliance will increase the dangers to their lives only embeds further the message sent when "normal" was used initially. "You'll be even more acutely different" speaks as much to people's social instincts as to their health-care concerns.

It makes sense for all who work with people to reflect on the language they use. Their word choice may be sending messages that are unintended but damaging. For people who do not have diabetes, unfortunate word choice can hurt feelings; for those who do have diabetes, words like "normal" can be devastating.

Another reason for my anger at that middle-aged man who spoke out at the support group meeting was that I recognized myself in him. After cooling down from my urge to strangle this unsuspecting man, I realized that I had not only been using the word NORMAL, but also had been thinking of myself and my diabetes in terms of NORMAL and ABNORMAL. I had been setting myself up as "different," "unhappy," "cursed," and a "have-not." My language had been sending the same damaging messages I found so offensive in others. I had been devastating myself and my own attempts at an effective diabetes management program. No wonder I was angry!

So, it makes even more sense for us with diabetes to rethink how we see ourselves and how we talk about ourselves and our diabetes. People without diabetes or without any particular awareness of how their language might hurt someone just don't know what they are saying and doing. They don't know any better. We do. Or we should. We need to rethink how we see ourselves. We should reconsider our notions of "normality." How different are we really? Who isn't different in some way? What does our being "diabetic" actually have to do with our place in society or our pursuit of happiness?

We might pay more attention to the language we use. By not using—and not buying into—words like "normal," we can create a more healthy attitude toward ourselves. Furthermore, we might even create a more healthy approach to our self-care and to the goals of our self-care. Plus—who knows?—we might even convert by example those without diabetes to a more caring attitude and a more careful use of language.

Exercise: Attitude Adjustment

Any member of a diabetes care team will tell you that exercise is "a crucial part" of the treatment of diabetes. Exercise is a "regimen"—something which should be"programmed" for "a maximum beneficial effect." It is another prescription—like insulin or a diet—to be taken daily: at about the same time each day for at least 25 to 30 minutes at a vigorous pace (70-80% of one's predicted heart rate: 220 minus one's age).

For me, this prescription had dealt me a cruel blow. Before I came out of the closet with my diabetes and sought up-to-date treatment of the disease, I used to love exercise. I used to revel in the games, the scores, the aesthetics, the pleasures, the pains, and the escape of exercise. For years, exercise and sports for me were clean and simple: clear-cut teams, rules, and results. They offered opportunities for fun, teamwork, and individual challenges. I have always played. I think that I was born with an athletic supporter on. Even now in my ripe old middle age I cannot resist choosing up sides and playing like my manhood was at stake. I have played organized and disorganized baseball, football, basketball, tennis, golf, racquetball, badminton, handball, and volleyball. I have been on wrestling and swimming teams. Some say that, if you have shirts and skins or different colored shirts and keep score, Raymond will play.

By the fall of 1983, soon after I had come out of the closet and had committed myself to up-to-date diabetes care, exercise had lost its delight. It had stopped being fun. It had become part of a regimen, a prescription, a "have-to." It had turned into work.

Exercise seemed like work for two reasons. First, it had to be done. It was an assignment. It was prescribed on a daily basis for a given period of time at a particular rate. It was associated with other regimens such as diet, blood tests, injections, and doctors' appointments. There just did not seem to be any choice: you did it or else.

It had become a task that I had to schedule into my life.

A second reason for exercise seeming like work was that it held little pleasure for me. As I was walking or running or cycling, I could not get it out of my mind the primary reason why I was exercising. With each slap of my feet on the pavement or each turn of the pedal, I was reminded that I have diabetes. "You have diabetes, you must exercise; you have diabetes, you must exercise; you have diabetes, you must exercise" ran through my head as I looked at my watch, counted the miles, or monitored the heart rate. Exercise had taken on the seriousness of being a life-or-death matter. So much for fun, delight, and the simple pleasures of competition.

What used to be a clear and simple escape to be enjoyed had been tainted by a disease which is neither clear nor simple. Rather than a simple pastime, exercise raised complex questions for which there are few—if any—clear-cut answers. How much insulin should I take if I play in the tennis tournament? What if the match goes three sets? What if it rains and the match is delayed? How much should I eat before I take off on my bicycle? How far in advance of the bike ride should I eat the extra food? What is the best food to eat? How long will it last? Did I miss that jump shot because my sugar is low?

No wonder it seemed easier to not exercise. All of those questions provided ample rationalization for staying in the easy chair and for not sweating. It is no mystery why something which used to be fun provoked anger. It also resulted in despair as I thought about how I used to feel about sports and exercise and how I began to feel. It was like a fall from purity and innocence. I felt like diabetes had stolen exercise from me.

I wanted it back. I have taken it back.

To get it back, I had to make some changes. First, I stopped being so rigid. I didn't do the same sort of exercising day in and day out. Some variety—like walking one day, running another, and cycling a third—relieved the tedium and thereby lessened the sense that exercise was a regimen. I walked another route. Also, I was not so compulsive about keeping track of time, distance, or my heart rate. Usually it takes me 40 to 45 minutes to walk three miles at a decent clip. Why insist on wearing a watch and staring at it? Thirty minutes on an exercise bike usually covers about twelve miles. Why stare at the odometer while pedaling away? I had been focusing on how slowly it was taking me to suffer through the ordeal. I made myself just pedal and sweat and pedal for 30 minutes and forget that pesky little dial which seemed to move more slowly than an inch worm. I focused on the scenery when jogging around the neighborhood.

A third thing I did was to distract myself from thinking so much about why I was exercising. I exercised with someone else. By carrying on a conversation while walking, I no longer contemplated the cruel injustices of Fate. (Plus, the conversation served to tell if I was overdoing it: if I cannot talk while exercising, I probably am going at it too hard.) I watched television. I set up the exercise bike in front of the TV and watched baseball or football games while pedaling away. This way I was having fun watching the game while doing my duty and not even noticing that I was pedaling my tail off. If a game wasn't on, I made myself think of something other than why I was working out. I made lesson plans up in my head or thought about how I would write the next chapter in my "great" American novel.

Another way that I took exercise back was to return to the challenge of it. One of the joys of exercise before it became treatment for diabetes had been the raw challenge of competition. I turned exercise into a set of goals: Can I run the three miles faster each time? Can I run farther this September than I did last year? How many laps can I swim in the pool before fatigue overwhelms me? Can I bicycle to work in a faster time than it would take me to drive my car? How much money am I saving by riding my bicycle to work rather than taking the car? I also used exercise as training for a special event like a road race or a tennis tournament. The running, the biking, or the pedaling wasn't for diabetes therapy; it was conditioning.

I also have used a reward system. If exercise is to be seen as a pain or a burden or anything nasty, why not compensate myself for enduring it? While I don't recommend a reward such as a dozen donuts, I worked for things I like. Once I bought myself a new hardbound novel after exercising every day for two weeks. But the reward need not be for a long-term performance. Sometimes it is a tall, ice cold diet Coke at the end of a run or an extra snack if I push myself an extra two miles. You can quite easily work up an elaborate system of positive reinforcements for a whole set of exercise activities. One summer, while working on losing some weight as well as a walking program, I used a credit system for earning a new basketball. (I took a lot of pleasure in the "sneaky" idea of making the reward another way for exercising.)

I reminded myself of my old friends—the games of youth. I asked myself why had I assumed that team sports were out or that the racquet sports didn't count. By thinking of exercise only in terms of diabetes therapy, I had forgotten that exercise can come in many forms. I didn't have to pedal a bicycle, walk or run miles, or swim laps. Games are legitimate: they are not useless just because you can keep score, play with friends, and have fun. Exercise need not be spelled s-u-f-f-e-r-i-n-g. Just because I happen to have diabetes does not mean that sport has to be left out of exercise. I pulled out my old sports equipment—a basketball, a softball, tennis balls, a racquetball racquet—and retired for a while the instruments of sweat and pain—running shoes, the exercise bicycle, sweatsuit, and my swimsuit. When exercise seems boring, painful, or solitary, I play sports. Games are fun, and they can accomplish the benefits of regimented exercise.

What I had was an attitude problem. Diabetes had not transformed sports and exercise into an ordeal. I had.

So, I adjusted my attitude. I took exercise back and made it fun again.

Insulin Reactions: Down the Black Hole

I DO NOT RECOMMEND insulin reactions.

In fact, I have had three types of "hypoglycemic episodes"—as the medical people call insulin reactions—and cannot recommend any of them.

The first type is common to most people who have diabetes. I call it the "stairway insulin reaction." It starts with a funny feeling in the pit of my stomach, in which a tiny hole seems to open up; that's when the funny feeling stops being funny. I start to perspire as hunger gnaws at the edges of the black hole. In anywhere from five to fifteen minutes, my energy slowly drains into the black hole. As the hole is gnawed wider and wider, all of my energy disappears and my sense of self begins to follow. The shakes sometimes try to consume my body. By then I have usually recognized what is going on and try to do something about it—eat about ten grams of easily absorbed simple sugar such as orange juice or honey.

Unfortunately, the will to do something is not matched by the ability to marshal the necessary resources. I get confused or disoriented. "Now what was I going to do? Oh yeah, get something to eat. Why? An insulin reaction. Food'll make my sugar go up." The body—"Whose body is that?"—refuses to move or is very sluggish. I may even stumble. The shakes and the sweats are industrial-strength by this time.

Even when I've eaten, the trip down the staircase goes on uninterrupted. I still stagger clumsily down that black hole in my stomach for up to thirty minutes, sometimes even after I have eaten something. It is not a pleasant journey.

The second type of insulin reaction is what I call the "whoosh reaction." With this reaction, I'll be playing tennis or working away or sitting in the lazy chair and all of a sudden—whoosh!—I'm at the bottom of the black hole. No funny feeling, no gnawing, no shakes, no sweating. I'm gone.

I discover myself far away yelling at my kids, chewing out students, and snarling at the world. Whoosh, I'm depressed. Sometimes "Why bother?" is camped out in my body, my brain, and my soul. Other times, I am mean and stubborn and surly. My nerves are on edge. I am irrational. I do not know why. It is as if someone has flipped a switch, and—whoosh!—I am at the bottom of the black hole. While certainly faster than the "staircase reaction," I cannot recommend the "whoosh reaction" either.

However, my least recommended reaction is the "silent reaction." It has no symptoms. There is no journey through a staircase of physical symptoms, nor is there the sense of hitting the bottom of a black hole. There are no symptoms: I don't feel a thing.

But the aftermath is substantial. "Silent reactions" occur most frequently during the night. When I wake up in the morning, the bed is soaking wet and smells like a locker room. My body feels like someone has been working it over with a baseball bat. My thighs and calves ache. I am exhausted.

"It couldn't be morning; I feel like I haven't slept a wink!...God, what awful nightmares I had!"

My mouth is dry, and the glucose test strip shows why. Even though my pre-bed glucose test was 130 and I had taken my insulin, my morning blood sugar is well over 400.

"Gee, I don't remember the chocolate cake that this represents," I moan.

The "silent reaction" has struck. I will pay for it all day. First of all, the sugar will not start down until well after lunch—if then. Second, I will be exhausted all day, dragging my rear end around like it was an iron anvil. Third, a full-blown evaluation of what caused the 400+ sugar will generate a guilt trip ("What did I do wrong?"), a loss of confidence ("Maybe it wasn't really an insulin reaction."), and the need to tinker with the diabetes management program ("Less insulin? More food? Less exercise? Sleep in the refrigerator? Buy a magic beeping watch?").

What is even more disturbing is that the "silent reaction" can strike while I am awake. I have had experiences when I have played three in tennis for about two hours and felt strong throughout the match. No staircase, no whoosh. No need to eat any of the emergency carbohydrates that I have in my bag (even though I should eat them regardless of how I feel). When I have gotten home, the evidence of the "silent reaction" becomes all too evident: terminal fatigue, excessive thirst, a headache, and a test strip so dark that the glucose monitor would scream if it could.

"Silent reactions" do not restrict themselves to vigorous activities like tennis or racquetball. I have been visited by them while working on a manuscript, assembling a bicycle, or doing anything else which requires concentration. I just do not feel the symptoms. The staircase and the whoosh are totally absent.

The black hole of the "silent reaction" is most frightening. Without feeling the symptoms, I am unable to treat them. When the body does not send signals—or when I miss the signals—insulin reactions go on uninterrupted.

I am at the mercy of my liver and the glucose that it stores. For some reason—such as excessive insulin, excessive exercise, too little food, drug interactions, or a combination of mysterious factors—the level of glucose in the blood is too low to "feed" the brain. Lower and lower the blood sugar goes, and the danger to my brain, my heart, and my central nervous system increases. (Because the brain is deprived, it sends signals to the heart and other organs that the body is in danger. First, the chemicals associated with fear-or-flight are pumped into the system. Then the brain starts shutting down, as does the rest of the system.) Fortunately, when the liver is working and contains stored glucose, my body will save itself by kicking in the stored glucose. (Drinking alcohol to excess can inhibit the liver's ability to save the body from an insulin reaction.) Unfortunately, the liver does not have the ability to cut off the glucose when the body is out of danger. The 400 + blood sugars result. Also, the liver may not have enough stored glucose to do the job. When the symptoms are not felt (due to medications such as beta blockers or the effects of long-term diabetes), or not recognized (easily done when asleep; involved in a hectic activity; or confused with symptoms of an illness, nervousness, or hunger), or when the liver does not serve as a lifesaver (pun intended), big problems can result—starting with unconsciousness, moving on to organ damage, and ending in possible death. Clearly, this black hole is the least recommended.

But what I *would* recommend is that we avoid as much as possible the staircase, the whoosh, and the silent insulin reaction. We can keep out of the clutches of the black holes. We can take our insulin as prescribed (types, amounts, and time). We can try to compensate for unexpected or unusual exertion by eating an extra snack. We can eat consistently by eating all of what we are allotted when we are due to have a meal. We can try to anticipate any changes in our meals, activities, stress, or routine and try to adjust our insulin and/or food. Just in case, we also should keep some simple sugar—candy, gel, tablets, or sugar packets—with us if we feel some symptoms of the black edging in on us. It's better to make a mistake ingesting a little too much sugar to prevent a possible reaction than to let yourself slip into an actual one.

Keep out of those black holes.

Affairs with Insulin Reactions

INSULIN REACTIONS and I have had a long and tortured history together.

In the beginning, I wooed insulin reactions as fervently as any lover. I had been taught at the onset of my diabetes that insulin reactions were a sign of good control. The "reasoning" was that, by keeping my blood sugar near 80-120, I was bound to suffer an insulin reaction. Any extra exertion, special stress, or missed snack would result in my dipping below 80 or so and experiencing an insulin reaction. In fact, a nurse once suggested that two to three reactions a week were desirable. I courted them without hesitation. I did not eat any sort of snack before, during, or after vigorous exercise. I tried to eat just a little less than I was allowed. I would ignore early symptoms of possible reactions to be sure that they were for real. What if I were wrong and it really wasn't a reaction? Taking something to eat would mess up my tight control and cut into my chances of living longer or living an "almost normal life."

But the romance did not last long. It became more and more difficult to court a lover who treated me so badly. On one occasion, I got into a horrendous fight with my father. What was I doing talking back to a father who believed that children were to be seen, not heard? It took Mom a long time to convince Dad that my unbelievable behavior was due to the diabetes. I kept away from him for several days.

On another day, when my blood sugar had gotten so low that I was nearly incoherent, I was found walking down the middle of the town's main street with cars and trucks barely missing me as I staggered right and left. People stared and gawked at that "strange little boy." For the next day or so, I had an awful headache and was exhausted. I felt like someone had beaten on my body with a hammer. Some kids at school talked quietly about me behind their hands the next day.

One summer night while at the Joslin Diabetes Camp in Massachusetts, I awakened to find myself in the camp's infirmary. A doctor had a needle in my arm, giving me some sort of glucose. I had no idea how I had gotten there. Apparently I had had a reaction while asleep and, because I was sleeping, was unable to treat it before it had gotten very bad. Unfortunately, my cabin companions did not hesitate to fill me in. I had gotten up in the middle of the night, stood on my bed, and started screaming. It had required several counselors to get me to the infirmary. Few in the camp restrained themselves from shaking their heads at me or saying something like, "Boy, you went crazy last night!" Everyone ensured that I had all of the details. The authorities kept me out of activities for the next two days.

But it took me a long time to develop a real disaffection for insulin reactions. It wasn't until I had left elementary school. As I entered junior high school and high school, my participation in organized sports became a main part of my life. Whether football, basketball, wrestling, baseball, or swimming, I played hard each and every season. I wasn't much of an athlete—I was never on a championship team—but I could have been better. I could have had a better opportunity. In football, for example, practices generally were organized so that calisthenics and drills were done before scrimmaging and final wind sprints. Invariably, I would get "low" just as the scrimmages would begin. It's pretty hard to impress the coaches when you have no energy and get disoriented. On many occasions, I forgot plays and missed blocking assignments. As a 135-pound guard trying to compete with guys built like Mack trucks, such lapses were not conducive to playing—let alone starting—on Saturdays. In swimming or wrestling, one cannot stoke up on calories before the big event and hope to perform to the best of one's ability.

How does one sprint 100 yards up and down the pool in free style with a lump of something in the stomach? In wrestling, I had to weigh in just before the evening matches. If I had eaten dinner or a snack for energy, making weight could have been a problem. Plus, if I had eaten and still made weight, I would have been completely ineffectual. Have you ever tried to be mobile, agile, and hostile with a lump in your stomach and another guy trying to throw you around and pin you? On the other hand, without the calories, an optimum performance was unlikely. At wrestling matches, my coach would frequently ask me why I did not have the speed or strength I had exhibited in practice.

Even when I was a starter—in basketball in junior high and in wrestling and swimming in high school—Dame Insulin Reaction had punished me. I still cringe with despair recalling when in big games or big matches I had run out of gas, suffered an insulin reaction, and let down my teammates. The game would be going on or the meet would be in full swing, and all of a sudden the symptoms would hit. How does one discreetly request a fifteen-to-twenty minute time-out to allow the sugar to kick in? Or say, "Excuse me. Can we delay the 115-pound match until I feel better?" Sure—when pigs fly.

By the second year of high school, I had had enough of insulin reactions. We parted with a serious alienation of affections. I developed absolute scorn for them. I would have nothing to do with them. It no longer mattered to me that they were supposed to reflect good control. I did everything and anything to avoid the embarrassment, the discomfort, the resulting fatigue, and the fears of not being able to perform at any time. I ate. I ate whenever I thought I might be playing ball or mowing a lawn or delivering newspapers or taking a test or delivering a speech. I ate regardless of the results of the blood sugar monitoring. Dame Insulin Reaction would not embarrass me or make me feel that hollow, impotent feeling in the pit of my stomach. I had had it with that "spaced out" feeling; I would not be sucked into that black hole. It felt better to have a high sugar than it did to have a low one. At that time in my life, it seemed better to risk the dangers of complications in the future than to suffer with the distress of reactions in the present.

Now—decades since the early torrid romance and years since our breaking up—insulin reactions and I have gone on to another phase of our relationship. The relationship no longer reflects the passions of desire or of hatred. I do not court insulin reactions, but neither am I excessive in my efforts to avoid them.

First of all, I have learned that insulin reactions are not symbolic of effective control. Their existence does not promise a longer or more "normal" life. Being low, I have learned, can be as dangerous—if not more dangerous—than being high. They can result in physiological damage—brain damage—and can cause the Somogyi effect, a rebound to sky-high sugars.

Second of all, I have developed a more rational response to the insulin reaction. I now know what the early symptoms are; I know how much to eat to keep the reaction from getting out of hand (approximately 20-30 grams of primary or simple carbohydrates such as 1/3 cup of apple juice, 1/2 cup of sweetened soda, three Lifesavers, or two packets of sugar). I know that it is better to eat something and be wrong about the onset of the reaction than it is not to respond quickly enough to actual symptoms. With more information about nutrition, I could handle more comfortably my need for energy while playing sports in school. If I had known about the staying power of proteins and about the existence of instant juice made from primary sugars, I might have been a starting guard all four years! But now I have a plan and an understanding of why that plan is essential.

I'd like to think that I have achieved a middle ground between my earliest passions for insulin reactions and my later scorn for them and reasonable sugar levels. However, I must admit that I have not de-programmed myself completely from the thinking that insulin reactions are not to be courted. On occasion, I still take a perverse pleasure in feeling one coming on: "Man, I'm being such a good boy! I must be keeping those sugars low." Sometimes I still hesitate to treat early symptoms because I distrust my judgment and fear that I am making the symptoms up in order to have something extra to eat. (I had a doctor accuse me of that once. I proved him wrong but still suffer with the accusation.) At other times I refuse to admit that I am having a reaction, because I would then have to admit that I have diabetes and that I was not able to master it.

But I am working on a better relationship with insulin reactions. Perhaps I could treat them like a distant relative: someone to know of, but someone who rarely visits.

Ketoacidosis in Pleasantville

KENNY WAS BORN early.

While a late-in-life baby for Mom and Dad, we kids were delighted. For more than six months, we had been jumping up and down in anticipation of a new brother or sister. As the eldest at 12 years old, I guaranteed that everything would remain on course when Mom had to go to the hospital. At 11, Holly and Jimmy promised to help cook and clean. Dad would be free to visit Mom and the baby in the hospital, to take a million pictures, and to give us full reports.

The whole family had been preparing for months. We kids learned how to use the washer and dryer, to cook meat loaf, and to sweep through the cleaning chores as a precision team. We practiced and practiced getting up early enough in the morning so that everything Mom had done would be completed by us kids before we had to catch the school bus.

We had become aces on the home front stuff. Ah, such pride!

The big day came—in fact, much too early in the day for my tastes. As Dad sped off to the hospital with Mom, our well-oiled, fine-tuned team cranked into action. For the first few days, all went well. The meat loaves rolled out of the oven; clean clothes instantly replaced piles of dirty clothes; we lingered at the bus stop waiting for the yellow chariot to pick us up. The nursery sparkled in anticipation of my newest brother's homecoming.

One day I even rode my bicycle into town to get some more insulin. I marched into the drug store, asked for a bottle of N.P.H. , and rushed to the grocery store for some ground beef for but another edition of Raymond meat loaf. I grunted up the hills trying to get home before Dad's return from the hospital. But he had beaten me by about 10 minutes. The house was in an uproar: Mom and Kenny would be home in just three days!

The uproar heightened each day. We all were so excited and so happy. But the night before the dynamic duo were due to arrive, I began to feel ill. I was pretty thirsty. I kept tanking up on water and was spending too much time in the bathroom. By the middle of the night, I was sick to my stomach, and by dawn I was vomiting. I had moved into the bathroom. Boy, I was exhausted and felt terrible.

"What a time for the flu! The very day that Kenny is coming home!"

Despite what I wanted to do, I had to slink off to bed. But things did not improve as the day went on. I no longer could show enthusiasm for living—let alone the homecoming festivities. All I wanted to do was sleep. But I kept trying to vomit. Then the stomach pain began. Oh, I wanted to die.

Dad became concerned. This seemed something worse than the flu to him. Then he noticed my breath: it smelled fruity and sickly sweet. He called the doctor. In a few hours, our family physician had me in the same hospital my mother had left just hours before.

"Ketoacidosis" was the diagnosis. My sugar was sky high. My body was breaking down body fat trying to fuel itself. For some reason, there was insufficient insulin in my body to utilize the food I had been eating. The waste by-products of this breakdown of fat were being dumped into my blood, my urine, my stomach, and my lungs. I was ill because my body was unintentionally poisoning itself. Immediate large doses of insulin allowed my body to feed without destroying its own tissue.

When I returned home in a few days, my introduction to Kenny was delayed. Dad wanted to know how I had gotten myself into such a fix. I protested that I had no idea. I swore that I had been taking my shots and that I had not been celebrating the birth of my brother by trying to eat all the candy in Westchester County. I assured him that I had not cheated on my diet. Who had time? The only time I had had a chance to get my hands on a Reese Cup was when I had pedaled into town to buy insulin. The very fact that I had bought insulin should prove to him that I had been taking the insulin.

Dad asked to see the insulin. It was not N. P. H. It was the wrong stuff! I had not checked to be sure that it matched what I had requested from the pharmacist. I had been taking a mixture totally unsuited for me, my diet, my life style, and my body. I couldn't understand how it had happened. Wrong insulin is one thing, but it seemed impossible that I could have slipped into so much trouble so quickly. That had not been a fun time. Ketoacidosis was definitely an unpleasant experience.

Dad began one of his famous—infamous?—"Now Son" lectures about how quickly young people can get into trouble with diabetes and about my needing to be more careful about what I was doing. He ended the entirely too long lecture with an admonition about being responsible. Then, as I tried to slide gracefully away, he winked and said, "You know you have a new brother. You have got to be around to help him grow up."

Victory #1: Retinopathy and the Laser

I COULDN'T UNDERSTAND IT.

For as long as I could remember, I had been seeking professional care by an ophthalmologist (a medical doctor who specializes in diseases of the eye) to keep track of my eyes. For decades, I had known that diabetes increased the chances for developing problems with my eyes, such as blurred vision, background retinopathy, and proliferative retinopathy as well as cataracts and glaucoma. So I had been careful—very careful.

In fact, I had seen an ophthalmologist regularly for years. There hadn't been any reports of developing problems. Since my last appointment, I hadn't noticed blind spots, "floaters," or cobwebs. There hadn't been any rapid shifts in my vision: no blurring, no distortion, no cloudiness, no sudden loss of ability to read, no slippage in peripheral (side) vision or night vision. Nothing had suggested that the long-feared problems had finally struck my eyes.

But, during a stay at a diabetes care unit for re-education and a medical checkup, I was asked to see an ophthalmologist who specialized in the vitreous (a clear, jelly-like material which fills the center of the eyes) and the retina (the "movie screen" on the back of the eye that focuses light entering the eye and sends the image to the brain).

The news wasn't good. After a thorough examination of both dilated eyes and a fluorescein angiography (photographs of the eyes' vessels are taken as dye passes through them), Dr. John Olson diagnosed background retinopathy in the left eye and proliferative retinopathy in the right eye. Because of high glucose levels and the diabetes, my left eye had grown small, abnormal blood vessels in the retina in an effort to improve impaired circulation. Unfortunately, because these vessels are "abnormal" (fragile and weak), they leak and break and leak blood or serum into the retina. The right eye was in worse shape. With proliferative retinopathy, the new vessels had grown on the retina's surface and into the vitreous. They could potentially cover the retina and obstruct vision, or bleed into the usually clear vitreous and obscure vision. They could also form scar tissue that could pull on the retina and separate it from the eye.

Dr. Olson calmly assured me that blindness was not a certainty. Drawings and printouts were used to explain what was happening and what would happen if nothing was done. He pressed for laser treatment—technically called pan-retinal photocoagulation. He expected the treatment to seal the abnormal vessels and to stop the progression of abnormal vessel growth onto the retina and into the vitreous. He recommended a series of two laser treatments for the right eye and careful, repeated observation for the left.

The laser treatments were scheduled for over the next two months to be done as an office procedure. For the first treatments, Dr. Olson dilated my right eye, gave me a local anesthetic, and positioned my head in a chin rest, He then shot the laser beams onto the retina, sealing off or destroying the leaking vessels. Both went without a hitch. Each treatment took about thirty minutes. I had to wear a patch for one day, and only once needed to take two aspirin for a slight headache. A month later, the follow-up checkup indicated that both procedures had gone well and that no further abnormal vessel growth was evident. No side effects were apparent: I did not notice any loss of peripheral vision, any night blindness, or anything else. Dr. Olson was delighted. He asked me to return in three months to be sure that the vessel growth and leakage had stopped. After a satisfactory checkup, he said I could return to sports activities such as tennis, racquetball, and running. But for now, he just didn't want any unusual pressure exerted on the eyes.

A few months later, apparent disaster struck. While playing a singles match of tennis one night, I noticed a small stream running down the middle of my vision. After rubbing my eyes and checking my glasses for something to account for the obstructed vision, I finally admitted to myself that the problem was with the interior of the right eye. I told Wayne, my opponent, that I could no longer continue to play, and headed home with a red opaque cloud that almost totally obscured the right eye's vision.

The late night telephone conversation with the sympathetic Dr. Olson told me it was probably a hemorrhage. He told me to discontinue the heart medication that I was taking to thin my blood and to make an appointment to see him after the hemorrhage had cleared enough so he could examine the retina and vitreous.

The examination a week later confirmed what Dr. Olson had suspected over the telephone: it was a hemorrhage; the scar tissue on the retina from the laser treatment had attached to the vitreous, which had pulled away from the retina. The tear had released blood into the eye and had obscured my vision. Dr. Olson said that the collected blood would eventually be absorbed, but he could not tell me how long it would take. He refused to attribute the hemorrhage to the strenuousness of the tennis match. He did not know if there would be any more hemorrhages. He would be neither optimistic nor pessimistic, but was certain that the hemorrhage was due to the scar tissue created by the laser treatment, not by diabetic retinopathy.

Having made an appointment to return a month later for a follow-up, I left Dr. Olson's office muttering about the irony of losing my vision from the treatment rather than from the retinopathy.

The ironic muttering rang hollow in the months that followed. Two months later, while working at a computer terminal, I suffered a second hemorrhage. (So much for the fear that the first hemorrhage had been brought about by pressure created during the exercise.) Three more months after that, a third hemorrhage struck while I was doing paperwork at my desk.

Each hemorrhage—with its unwelcome stream of blood, its obscuring red cloud, and its very slow absorption—provoked an emotional cycle of anger, despair, and resignation. Repeatedly I asked myself, "Won't it ever end?"

But the cycle did end.

Eighteen months after the original appointment and eight months since the last hemorrhage, the checkup with the ophthalmologist proved encouraging. Dr. Olson had trouble finding the abnormal vessels in the left eye. The hemorrhage in the right eye was clearing; the vitreous had fully separated from the right eye's retina—a natural occurrence as we age—which meant that there was little chance of another hemorrhage developing because of the scar tissue.

More importantly, little or no change had occurred in either eye. Apparently the retinopathy had been checked by the laser treatments and by the greater attention to the monitoring of my blood sugars.

I made an appointment for a regular checkup in six months and left the ophthalmologist's office feeling for the first time in two decades that I just might not have to be blind.

Laser Treatment:
A Patient's Perspective

WHEN THE DOCTOR told me that I needed laser treatments on my eye, I was afraid. Despite his patient efforts to convince me not to worry, I was not comforted. Would it hurt? What could go wrong? What were the possible consequences? I kept thinking, "The doctor is a respected expert, but has he ever had laser surgery?" The very words "laser surgery" made me shudder.

After three extensive treatments, I now know that I needn't have worried so much. Both experiences were among the easiest medical procedures I have ever been through. In fact, the most difficult part was the worrying.

When the doctor explained the process, it seems to me he described it in terms of the greatest discomfort that could be expected. Fortunately, my experiences didn't come close to what he had described. And I am the type who passes out just driving through a hospital zone, whose blood pressure goes sky high at the mere mention of the word "doctor," and who takes bodyguards whenever he goes for anything even remotely resembling a medical procedure.

Step #1 involved instilling drops into the eye in order to dilate it. I really did not like this. I can't stand anything in my eye—to say nothing of three sets of drops!

Step #2 demanded the very nerve-racking process of waiting for the eye to dilate. Boy, the things my mind thought up during those 15 to 20 minutes! What a job trying to act casual while my imagination ran wild!

Step #3 required an injection to ensure that the eye to be treated did not move during the actual laser use. To be frank, this step turned out to be the most uncomfortable in the whole process. The doctor injects the eyelid with an agent to numb the muscle. It pricks momentarily. (In fact, the prick hurt the most the first time. The second time I must have been more relaxed—if relaxation is ever possible—because I barely noticed it.) But, since the eyelid has so few nerves, it did not really hurt very much either time. Step #4 was another waiting period. During the first experience, it was a time for becoming tense; the second time, I just talked with my bodyguard.

The actual laser treatment—step #5—required my moving into the special room. It appeared dark, small, and full of equipment. But, of course, it is tough recalling details when you are wasting your energy being afraid. The doctor placed me in a chair, had me rest my chin on a mask-like frame, and inserted a contact lens onto the eye. (He told me about the lens; I couldn't feel more than a little pressure.) After loosely clamping my head so it would not move, the doctor moved the laser into position.

"Let me line this up first," he commented. I stopped breathing.

"Please try not to move your head." I held onto the table for dear life.

"Don't worry; you won't be able to move the eye." I counted the clicks some machine was making.

"It looks good." Fifteen minutes or so had passed, and I was starting to wonder when he was going to start the treatment. Then the doctor was telling me that it was all over.

"Take aspirin or Tylenol should you develop a headache. Leave the eye covered for about twenty-four hours." I could not believe that he was putting a patch over the eye.

I started to breathe again. I released his table. A mile-wide grin creased my once gloomy face. My bodyguard and I left the office and went out to get a cup of coffee.

"Nothing to it." I beamed as passersby stared at my impressive bandage. If they only knew how easy it had been. A day later I took the patch off and went back to work—using both eyes. I never noticed even any temporary side effects such as the loss of night vision or the loss of any peripheral vision.

The only discomforts I have ever experienced from laser treatments have resulted from the anxieties about how it would be, the injections to immobilize the eye to be treated, and once when I developed a headache the evening after a treatment. (I had refused to take aspirin because the first time it had been so painless.)

Isn't it silly how people worry? Would you believe that during visits to the doctors' offices I have observed or heard all sorts of anxieties of people while they are awaiting a laser treatment? If they only knew the truth! The worst part is the fear.

Now they know.

Victory #2: Control and the Kidneys

"AH, WHAT A RELIEF!"

With the results of the creatinine clearance test back from the laboratory, I sighed in relief. Despite decades of somewhat-less-than-effective control of my diabetes, my kidney function was within the normal range. The laboratory analysis of my urine collected over twenty-four hours revealed that the amount of waste (creatinine) filtered through the kidneys and spilled into the urine was within normal range. Low normal—but still normal.

I had been worrying for some time over my kidney function. I knew all too well the threats that long-term diabetes brought to the kidneys: infections, hardening of the small kidney arteries, decreasing ability to filter out wastes. I knew that high glucose levels in the blood damage the small blood vessels in the kidney. When these vessels are damaged, the kidney cannot filter out wastes and toxins. So, each time I went for my regular appointment I expected the doctor to report that I had reached stage three in the development of kidney disease (nephropathy): large amounts of protein in my urine and fluid retention by my body. Visions of dialysis and a kidney transplant frequently had been weighing heavily on my mind.

So, for the latest test, I had dutifully collected my urine for twenty-four hours and fearfully awaited the results of the creatinine clearance's measurement of my kidney function. Thankful for the unexpected results, I went home determined to improve the control of my diabetes by monitoring my sugars and adjusting my insulin. I wanted to show my gratitude for this good fortune and to take advantage of the second chance. For well over a year, I did work very hard. I focused on exercise and diet as well as on monitoring my sugars, seeing the doctor, and adjusting my insulin.

But that hard work had not always resulted in the sincerely desired control. Insulin reactions, unusual stress, unrecognized infections, and overzealous eating produced blood sugar numbers too often in the 300s, 400s, and above. The introductions of a new diet, new insulins, a new injection schedule, a variety of medications, and a different work schedule played havoc with the desired control. This havoc, in turn, led to despair over the possibility of my effectively maintaining control and sometimes to my abandoning the program for balancing diet, exercise, insulin, and medication. For over a year, it had seemed that there were as many blood sugars in the 300s and 400s as there were in the 80-to-180 range.

As I looked back over the year's efforts at improved control, I was unhappy with the difference between what I had set out to accomplish and what I had done. Holding out little hope for encouraging results, I reluctantly submitted to another creatinine clearance test.

Surprise! Two days later, the lab report documented a significantly improved kidney function.

This time there was more than a mere sigh of relief: I celebrated with a whoop! Even with the less-than-satisfactory efforts for improved control, I had been able to improve my kidney function. It was not only a victory for my kidneys, but also for the hopes that something can be done by working at managing my diabetes.

Impotence: The Case of Careless Words

THAT BEAUTIFUL SPRING afternoon turned out to be Black Monday.

Despite the flowers' stretching to the warm sun, the gentle breezes' loving caress of the budding trees, and the fluffy clouds' flow to the east, I was suffering with the flu. In fact, I had ached and throbbed throughout what had been a beautiful weekend and had gone to the university infirmary seeking relief. I ended up with something which would haunt me for decades.

Judy and I had been married just that last August in 1968 and had begun graduate school in September. By that spring we still were basking in the golden glow of the honeymoon period. We had plans; Judy would earn her M.A.; I would earn an M.A. and a Ph.D.; we would get teaching positions; we would raise a family and devote ourselves to the pursuit of happiness and the rest of the American Dream.

A doctors' careless words certainly dimmed the glow of our honeymoon period and tarnished our vision of our once-golden prospects.

After the infirmary doctor took vital signs, diagnosed that I had the flu, and perfunctorily prescribed the usual treatments, he turned down a dark path.

"Oh, you have diabetes."

"Yes."

"How long have you had diabetes?"

"Eighteen years."

"Are you married?"

"Yes."

"How long have you been married?"

"Almost eight months."

"Well, you had better hurry up and have children. Impotence is a serious problem with those who have diabetes. . . . Have a good day."

The doctor whisked out of the examination room, leaving me stunned and sputtering. My flu was long forgotten. It seemed ironic that I had thought that the aches and pains of the flu were interfering with my concentration on the graduate work.

Those careless, unexplained words would haunt me for years: ". . . you had better hurry up and have children. Impotence is a serious problem with those who have diabetes."

I never repeated those words aloud. I kept them to myself and worried. The gentle flow of our lives took on a sense of urgency. The pace of my pursuit of the graduate degrees escalated to a fever pitch. I was driven by the urge to get on with my life and with our dreams. Our lovemaking wasn't the same. I seemed to be in a hurry. My sexual appetite seemed insatiable. I was young. The dark specter of impending impotence seemed to sit on the edge of our bed waiting to tap me on the shoulder and to end our intimacy. The careless words had turned me suddenly into an insensitive, inadequate man who feared being even more inadequate.

The impact of those careless words did not diminish as time passed. To the contrary, as we passed through the stages of our lives, I became more and more anxious. When Judy finished her M.A. and went to work, I would rush home early from the graduate library with champagne and steak to greet her. We would make love on the living room floor, and she would tease me about being in such a rush all the time. No doubt she wondered what had happened to a person she had known for over six years. When I finally finished my class work and took a temporary instructorship at a college, I began to press her to stop taking the pill and to have children. She was not sure she wanted children. With my instructorship due to run out after two years, she certainly was not anxious to leave her job, to get pregnant, and to create any more major responsibilities for either of us. Our life was not exactly a model of stability.

The more insistent I became about starting a family the more distant we were with each other. We began to argue. The pressure kept building. I directed all of my energies to my work. I spent more and more time in my office, trying to exercise some control over some part of my life by publishing. If I wasn't working, I was coaching a football team at the junior high school, playing football on a faculty intramural team, or infrequently working on my doctoral dissertation. This was nearly five years after that spring visit to the infirmary.

Now Judy and I have been married for more than two decades (yikes!). We did have children—two sons—eight years after we were married. My diabetes has been with me for more than 36 years. I have had only two very temporary experiences with impotence. But we certainly have suffered with the idea of it. I believe that its haunting possibility nearly ended our marriage, created enormous conscious and unconscious pressures within me, and generally affected every part of my life.

I still worry about impotence, but I am not in as much of a panic as I was before.

One reason for my panic somewhat subsiding is that I now know more about impotence and diabetes. After all those years of anxiety and ignorance, I finally faced the disruptive issue that those careless words had introduced into my life. I asked qualified people questions and sought reliable reading materials. It was amazing how much relief there can be in a little information! I first learned that a great deal of impotence is psychological. The more one worries about it the greater the chance for problems. It occurred to me that one does not have to have diabetes to have psychological anxieties about sexual dysfunction. Also it became obvious that my worrying about impotence and diabetes was more of a threat than the actual diabetes.

I also learned about the physical causes for impotence. If a man has had diabetes for a number of years, the high blood glucose levels can result in nerve damage (neuropathy) and/or disease of the blood vessels (arteriosclerosis). Because of nerve damage, a person isn't as able to be as responsive to stimulation. The circulatory or vascular problems inhibit the flow of blood to the penis and thereby can prohibit an erection. Even particularly elevated blood sugars at a given time may result in impotence. I also learned that certain medications, such as those for high blood pressure, can cause impotence.

This information admittedly brought mixed lessons. The first physical cause did not represent a direct threat—knock on wood—because recent nerve induction tests revealed I had no apparent nerve damage. The second and fourth causes were of more concern because of my adventures with heart and artery disease and my blood pressure medications. The third, blood sugar levels, seemed one cause more easily corrected. Even if I were to suffer from three of the main physical causes, I could still turn to new improvements in drug therapy, implants, a variety of by-pass procedures, avoiding high and low blood sugars, and other research being conducted.

Furthermore, impotence is not a certainty for men with diabetes. While the figures differ, it seems that men with diabetes have only a 50% greater chance of impotence than their counterparts without the disease and that by the time the man with diabetes is older than 50, he only has a 50% chance of being afflicted with impotence. While not totally comforting, such odds did indicate to me that I do have a good chance of escaping the impotence that the doctor with his careless words had virtually guaranteed me in 1969.

Another reason the panic is not so pervasive is that I am nearly into middle age. (Hah, I am middle-aged!) We have our two sons, are grateful for them, and will have no more children. I am older and considerably (somewhat?) more mature. As a result, Judy and I are more communicative, more open, and therefore less susceptible to the pressures of cultural stereotypes. I am more secure in our relationship and feel that our intimacy is based on more than my sexual performance.

To be sure, I still worry about impotence. But it does not haunt me as it did before and I am no longer in a panic. I have had a full life without it so far and now know enough about it to prevent total despair over the prospects.

I wish I had not succumbed to that doctor's careless words so many years ago. The cost was too high.

The Books and S-E-X

I WAS HAVING A "potential problem"—actually, a real problem—that I thought might be connected with my diabetes. I went to the library seeking information from recent books because of the delicate nature of the "problem." I wanted to read and know more about the basics before I launched into a nervous and embarrassing discussion with someone about sex in general and impotence in particular. On occasion, I had been unable to get an erection and, on another occasion, had been unable to sustain an erection. (Actually, I was hoping that the books would take care of the "problem" and that I would not have to talk to any doctor, nurse, or counselor about my problem with "s-e-x.")

I was surprised to find so many books on diabetes in the public and the university libraries. However, to my dismay, some of the books were not as helpful as I had hoped. Two hadn't included anything about s-e-x, although one claimed to focus on living with diabetes and the other on having diabetes and having fun. It just seemed to me that s-e-x had something to do with living and having fun. Two other books offered more. One, in about five pages, answered the following questions: Will my diabetes cause sex problems? What can you do about impotence that is mainly psychological? What about physical impotence in men with diabetes? Does diabetes cause male sterility? While the answers were not exhaustive, they did deal with female and male sexuality, did suggest possible causes for physical and psychological sexual problems and referred readers to other sources. In about twelve pages devoted to sexuality and diabetes, the other covered three main topics: marriage and sexuality, female responses, and male impotence. Their coverage seemed more detailed and more candid.

I feel very lucky to have found these two books. I wonder what might have happened if I had had access to only the first two books. How would I have reacted if the second two had not been in the local library? Might not a shy, an insecure, or an easily embarrassed person with diabetes and with sexual problems decide not to pursue it any further? Might one assume that he or she were the only ones with diabetes who had sexual problems? Isn't it possible that one might conclude, because impotence was not mentioned in books by doctors, that sexual problems are not related to diabetes?

If people with diabetes are left to their own ignorance, half-knowledge, or fears regarding such vital parts of living as s-e-x or depend upon sources which are not helpful or incomplete, they can end up in big trouble. If it is a physical problem, they could wait so long to do something about it that they could end up being beyond help. If it is a psychological problem, they could begin a downward spiral of depression and dysfunction which could take years of therapy to escape.

I was lucky. A number of authorities were available and I was persistent enough to keep looking until I found some people who acknowledged the existence of the problem, recommended some causes and effects, and cited other more detailed sources of information. Armed with the awareness that I wasn't the only person with diabetes in the annals of medical history who had questions about sexuality and diabetes and with some basic information, I felt more comfortable about pursuing the issue with the doctor and other people with diabetes.

Unfortunately, I suspect that others are not so lucky. Whether sex, headaches, or eye problems, I am afraid that some people with diabetes have sought help unsuccessfully from inadequate libraries or uninformed people. They, then, may have given up their quest, assumed that they were the only ones with such problems, and have suffered alone.

I was lucky because by accident I learned that not all sources are complete and/or accurate. I also learned that I might have to be persistent in order to get full or reliable information.

I was lucky because I learned that impotence usually results from problems in four areas: vascular (impaired blood circulation), neurological (nerve damage), psychological (decreased desire, stress, anxiety), or the side effects of drugs. I also learned that a great deal of research has been conducted regarding sexual dysfunction and diabetes. Not only was I not alone—if, indeed, I were suffering from impotence—but many opportunities were available for treating the problem. I could try other medications to treat my elevated blood pressure; counseling might alleviate my anxieties; vasoactive drugs are available to aid circulation. I even learned that there were penile prostheses that could be surgically implanted.

I was even luckier. Once I had all this information, my "potential problem" disappeared.

Being a Parent with Diabetes

My sons suffer with my diabetes. They have suffered with my disease for longer than they have existed.

Eric and Bryan almost were not conceived. For nearly two decades, I had carried around the burdensome assumption that diabetes was strictly an hereditary disease. When diagnosed, I recall the doctor's careful questioning of my father and mother about who in their respective families had had diabetes. Their inability to come up with anyone was met with pressing interrogations: someone had to have had diabetes; someone was responsible for passing it along. Throughout the diabetes education program that my parents and I went through in 1955, we were taught that there was an extremely high probability that I would pass the disease onto my children. At that point, my parents were more distraught about this than I. But, even for a nine-year-old, the message was clear—the "curse" was passed on; children of "diabetics" were "diabetic." As I grew up, the dimensions of having diabetes became more and more evident to me. As I discovered women and began dating, the currently held theories on how a person got diabetes took on greater significance. The idea of passing on diabetes grew into a concern.

Who would willingly pass on a life with diabetes—a life with a disease that requires restricted diets, insulin injections, and ominous complications? It did not seem like a good idea to me. Unfortunately, I had wanted to have children for a long time. I had wanted to love them selflessly and without reservation. They represented a major portion of my personal American Dream—the pursuit of happiness. But I was not willing to trade my pursuit of happiness for the risk of subjecting my children to a disease that I had not found easy to live with or very comforting.

Who would willingly bring children into a less than perfect world when the prospective father has at best an uncertain future and at worst no future at all? I had been the eldest son in a family whose husband/father/provider had been killed in an accident at age 38. The effects of his death had been devastating to my mother, my sister (aged 13), my brother (4), and me (15). The emotional trauma from the loss far surpassed the genuine financial difficulties. While I rationally knew that no one's life is guaranteed, it seemed an unreasonable and unloving thing to expose children to a repetition of my family's history. Having children just did not seem a good idea.

For eight years my wife and I wrestled with the children-or-no-children dilemma. The struggle nearly poisoned our lives. Eric was born in 1976: an "accident" to me, a marriage-saving solution to Judy. Bryan was born in 1978: a conscious decision by Judy and me that the love and happiness that Eric had brought into our lives outweighed the risks involved.

However, in spite of my devotion to them, my sons have suffered with my diabetes since their conception. Mostly, they have suffered with the personality of a father with diabetes who goes through the gloom-and-doom moods of waiting for disaster. When something goes wrong, I get depressed. Eric and Bryan easily sense my mood and frequently succumb to it themselves. I can turn their beautiful summers into dark, stormy days. They suffer the irrationality that comes with Dad's low blood sugars and insulin reactions. They are bewildered when I seem incoherent, weak, and disoriented. Who can blame them when they wonder what had happened to their usually exuberant father? "It's his diabetes" hardly relieves them. Doctor's appointments do not delight their breadwinner. I worry about the money demanded by the constant medical care. When modern medical science fails to come through with good news or a miracle solution, they overhear bitter remarks about the low cost-benefit ratio involved with medicine. They hear me complain about four shots a day, wish that I could drink a case of beer, and lament that my life is full of scheduled tests, shots, meals, and appointments.

Ah, what of their "lamb white days"? How are they to enjoy young and easy days under the apple boughs when their father cannot sing in his chains? They suffer with and share my gloomy despair, rising anger, and waning hope.

This suffering is not my imagination working overtime. Eric and Bryan hover around the kitchen table when I monitor my blood sugar in the morning. When the strip darkens, they literally flee because they know that it is going to be a dark morning. They are certain that an explosion is coming in short order.

They hide when they are enjoying their ice cream, candy, or cake. One evening we were watching television together, but their backs were turned toward me. They were trying to conceal bowls of vanilla ice cream and chocolate chip cookies. They knew that "Daddy shouldn't eat sugar." They were afraid of hurting my feelings and felt guilty enjoying their desserts. When I am particularly enjoying a meal or a beer, my two sons have been known to assure me that they wouldn't tell Mommy.

One day Bryan, the youngest, said, "I wish you didn't have to take shots." Then, after pausing, he muttered, "I sure hope I don't get diabetes!" On another occasion, the older Eric reassured me, "You are a good father, even if you do have diabetes." Just last week, the oldest asked me to guess what his first wish would be if he had magical powers. When I said I couldn't guess, he said, "That you did not have diabetes."

While unintended, the messages seem clear. First, I have established an uncomfortable, unhealthy atmosphere in our home. Frequently things are dark, ominous, frightening, and different from the homes of "normal" families. Anxiety is ever present in me and is passed onto the children.

Second, because of my responses to my diabetes, I have two children—and frequently a wife—who walk on eggshells around me and my handling (or non-handling) of my disease. Rarely does spontaneity run free in our home. How this or that will affect Dad's mood or schedule or diet or blood sugar is considered before it is planned or done. Tip-toeing through life hardly seems appropriate for childhood.

Third, what kind of model is a parent who acts like a peevish child? Children learn more from observing adults and parents than they do from all the lectures in the world. The sort of behavior that I have shown them throughout their lives only can teach them things which will make their future lives miserable. Who wants to play with, work with, or associate with someone who is so touchy? As far as Eric and Bryan know, that is "adult" behavior; their Daddy does it.

Fourth, they focus as nearly as much as I do on my diabetes. Although diabetes comprises a relatively small portion of my life, I have centered on my perceptions of my life on diabetes. Rather than choosing my writing, my teaching, my athletics, or various life experiences, I select what is wrong. Neglecting what I can do, I emphasize what I cannot do. Limitations because of diabetes seem more important than the things that I can do well. They see me as a "diabetic" because indirectly I have insisted upon it. Also, I have shown them that what one lacks outweighs what one has.

Fifth, I have influenced their perceptions of food, needles, doctors, exercise, and everything at all connected to living with (against?) diabetes. They see the world from a "diabetic" perspective. While much of that perspective could be healthy and could contribute to a longer, more sensible life span, it also can dampen a child's enthusiasm for living. Children usually do not—and should not have to—invest themselves in long-term benefits. Life should not be lived defensively. Joy! Surprise! Crazy days! Howling in delight! Why not? Sure! Go for it! Exercise and food can be fun; doctors are people who can be partners in a life of wellness; modern medical science need not be seen as big business or as experiments in technology.

Finally—heaven forbid!—what has been my effect upon them if, indeed, Eric or Bryan is in that very small percentage of those who develop diabetes? What have I set them up for? Regardless of living in general, what about living with diabetes when they have spent their entire lives watching a semi-crazy person battle the disease by ignoring it, by attacking it in an unrelenting frenzy, or by slumping into complete despair? I would not wish them to live their lives in any of these ways. Why do I? Besides not exactly healthy for me, not one of these approaches to diabetes represents a worthwhile or wholesome prospect for them.

More than anything, I wish for Eric and Bryan to have their chances to pursue happiness. They have been *my* happiness. I believe that my diabetes has contributed to my valuing them as the treasures they are. Because of the disease, I am sensitive to the precariousness of life. With this heightened sensitivity, I tend to enjoy the boys, to spend as much time with them as possible, and to work hard at being a good father for them.

If they do not develop diabetes, they still deserve a model which allows them to develop without extraordinary doses of despair, slanted perceptions of everything from food to doctors, and heightened apprehensions about just living. They deserve a model of living life as a process of wellness. If they do develop diabetes, they will need a model which allows them to live with the disease. They deserve not to be burdened with decades of ancient attitudes, techniques, and expectations dealing with diabetes. They should be prepared for living a positive, aggressive life with diabetes.

I should not wait. The model is necessary now. If I wait, it will be too late for the model to do any good. Eric and Bryan will not believe the model if I don't live it for as long as they can remember. They will question its authenticity if it appears only for them.

Sure, I am human. Certainly, getting diabetes is not one of the wishes usually asked of the genie in the magic lamp. But I cannot bear for my sons to suffer with my diabetes, now or down the road. When they suffer, I suffer. I need to be a better parent. I can be a better parent by approaching my diabetes as a process of working toward wellness.

How?

I try to be a parent—a loving father—rather than a parent with diabetes. The disease is a major part of my life, but it need not dominate my children's lives nor shape how I treat them. I try to not let it dominate what I talk about or what I do. It's important that I think I am a parent, not a parent with diabetes. If I can do that, then perhaps I will be able to act like a parent naturally.

Second, when the diabetes does have a part in our lives together, I try to educate them about the disease. Of course, that requires that I know as much as possible about it. Nevertheless, I think they benefit if they know what is and what is not a by-product of the diabetes. When, for example, I endure an insulin reaction and do or say something I regret, I believe it is important to do two things. One is to apologize for whatever I have done. The other is to explain what the reasons are for that behavior. Furthermore, when I talk to them about my diabetes, I work at presenting my management efforts as a making of choices, as doing things which will help me better enjoy them and life, and as a positive challenge. Rather than trying to prevent the terrible catastrophes of complications, I work for wellness and a more fulfilling life.

Also, I work on not turning the diabetes into the scapegoat. To suggest to Eric and Bryan that I would be perfect if it weren't for the diabetes does not serve them well. Even if they don't see how ridiculously untrue that idea is, they need to know that parents are human and are not perfect. (That certainly will relieve the pressure on them when they are parents.) Furthermore, it keeps us from turning diabetes into the terrible thing which has ruined an otherwise per-fect existence.

Third, I try not to be so self-centered. Sure, living with diabetes is no picnic. But the diabetes is *my* disease, not theirs. I am a better parent for my sons if I am more mature as I wrestle with managing my disease. Having a tantrum over a blood sugar, a doctor's ap-pointment, or the rising cost of disposable syringes isn't very useful for anyone. Pouting or grousing just because I have to do something serves little purpose. I try to talk more about my management pro-gram: tell them that shots don't usually hurt, that it's not really that much of a problem to monitor my blood glucose, or that I don't have an emotional investment in what I can or cannot eat. When I do scream, pout, grouse, or complain, I try to take the time later to explain that most of it isn't that big of a deal, that I was just letting off some steam.

Another strategy for becoming a better parent is to do things which show that diabetes doesn't dominate their or their father's life. For me, this includes a spontaneous day trip, a visit to the ice cream store for a "forbidden" treat, or a day without glucose monitoring. (It is important not to lament the damage I might be doing or worrying aloud about the diabetes.) If not done to ex-tremes, the boys can see that Pop's able to do what he wants and that he is, indeed, in control and can make choices about how he will live.

Finally, I remind myself that I love Eric and Bryan and that that is the most important thing I can do for them. By remembering that and assuring myself that I am doing the best I can do with the diabetes and with raising them, I am easier on myself. By not spending so much time lashing myself, I think I have a better chance of being a better parent.

A Response to
"Being a Parent with Diabetes"
by Maggie Duvall

My Daddy had diabetes. I have diabetes. I love my Dad. I'm glad he had the courage to have me.

My Dad got diabetes when he was 18 years old. He had diabetes when I was born. I thought everybody's dad took shots in the morning. I thought Clinitest tablets and a test tube in a glass were on the back of everyone's john. I knew my Dad loved me.

When I got older, I knew other dads didn't have diabetes. I knew they didn't take shots every morning. I thought my Dad was very brave. I knew my Dad loved me.

When I hit the "double digits," I began to notice that my Dad would sometimes be "moody." He had his first hemorrhage then. My sister got diabetes then. The moods would leave, but they would come back. I did not fear the moods, and I did not always understand them. I did not know if the moods were different from the "norm" nor did it matter. I gave Dad space until he got better. I knew my Dad loved me.

By the time I hit my late teens, I knew more about my Dad and his "moods." I knew that they were mostly related to his diabetes. I also knew of his anger and frustration as it related to diabetes. I knew of his hostility toward doctors and pharmacists and insurance companies. I knew my Dad loved me.

Only when I too became a parent did I appreciate even more of my Dad's many qualities. Some of those qualities were evident because he lived so many years with diabetes—some just because of his uniqueness, whatever the source. I was able to see and love and hopefully appreciate his humanness. He had never been a larger-than-life, unapproachable kind of Dad. I had seen him suffer, then recover. He passed to me his strength by the example he set—by the way he lived his life. By the way he loved me.

Mike, I know that your sons Eric and Bryan are lucky boys. The fact that you have diabetes may, for them, turn out to be more of a blessing than a curse. I'm sure that they know that their dad loves them—and that's about all that really matters.

Parenting a Child With Diabetes

BEING A PARENT is tricky business. As people bring a child into this everchanging world, they suffer for and with that child. Parents want it all for the son or daughter. They want the child to "have it better than they did." They want their boy or girl to be "happy." They want the person that they brought into existence to be "successful."

This parenting business makes extraordinary, seemingly contradictory demands upon mere mortals. They are expected to love deeply and to discipline rigorously, to applaud accomplishments and to make demands, to protect and to shove out of the nest, to be truth-givers and to nurture truth-seekers, to be models and to be humans, to teach them to be scholars and to train them to be athletes, to foster conscientious community members and to insist upon unique individuals.

These severe demands are to be met in a world that often is baffling. The rapid advancement of technology, the increasing pace of daily life, and the changing face of social structures make for a world that is different from one day to the next. Today's truth was yesterday's dream and will be tomorrow's ancient history. Once essential jobs can be obsolete and nonexistent in a blink. School systems teach concepts that become outdated the moment they are presented. Day-in and day-out newspapers report events that may or may not be true and that may or may not change the job market, the country's leaders, or the cost of gasoline. Indeed, being a parent is a tough, uncertain task.

Then add to the job the complex dimensions involved when the son or daughter has diabetes.

First, diabetes adds to the already seemingly endless list of responsibilities for a parent. For a parent who has a child with diabetes, the list is lengthened with the duties of overseeing and helping to manage diet, exercise, glucose monitoring, insulin doses, insulin injections, medical appointments, and all the rest. These new tasks are the easiest to perform, although they are not easy.

The parent has to learn so much about the disease: the good news, the bad news, the techniques, the variables, the developments, the numbers, the biology. Without formal medical training, parents can find themselves discussing ketones, insulin pumps, carbohydrates, the Somogyi effect, or peripheral vascular disease. Through reading, instruction, or experience, they have to develop a working knowledge for helping to balance food, exercise, stress, and insulin. They have to serve as a storehouse of information and to ensure that enough medical supplies are on hand. They have to provide the money for buying the syringes, the insulin, the special foods, the test strips, and all the other stuff. They have to be prepared to step in at any moment to give shots, to help treat an insulin reaction, or to set up essential appointments.

Second, the parents of someone with diabetes find themselves serving like foremen on a cattle drive. While the son or daughter is responsible for doing the work involved in managing the disease, the parent-as-foreman oversees the jobs. They check procedures, offer suggestions, and step in with required help. Sometimes the offspring act like wayward steers. They wander off. They neglect to monitor, to inject, to eat, to exercise, or to remember that they have diabetes. The parent-as-foreman rides into the underbrush to nudge the wayward ones back into safety. Sometimes the methods are gentle, sometimes forceful and authoritative.

A third role in parenting a child with diabetes involves the delicate process of providing emotional support and counsel. Children in general represent formidable challenges for advising. From the first days they speak until the day they have their own children, kids ask peculiar questions and seek (and frequently reject) the opinions of their elders. Oh, the topics and problems could keep a full-time professional psychiatrist busy. Parents face inquiries about Santa Claus, the sky's color, politics, sex, religion, the meaning of life, and other such topics for light conversation.

Of course, such questions are not in isolation. Parents have their own questions and sometimes don't have answers for themselves, let alone for their children. They can feel pressured to know answers or to be "right." Furthermore, parents have their own problems which can confuse the issues being considered. They can become emotionally involved in situations that require objective evaluation and recommendations. Parents also have to serve as disciplinarians for the children they are trying to advise. The people who set rules, curfews, and allowances frequently have difficulties being accepted as credible or trusted counselors. The person who assigns chores and who can get involved in a titanic struggle with offspring over authority and freedom does not come across as "friendly" to a son or daughter.

Plus, parents and children live together. How often have parents found themselves doing things that they have advised their children not to do? Battles over territory seem standard operating procedure. Arguments over the television, the family car, and personal space can inhibit the free flow of ideas. Choices of music, clothing, and food have been known to disrupt the most peaceful of families and interfere in heart-to-heart talks.

To have to mix the uncertain terrains of diabetes into these characteristically difficult parental responsibilities of providing emotional support and counseling is to make the successful fulfillment of the tasks seems nearly impossible.

Children with diabetes face compounded problems in living. As children without diabetes grow up, they exercise their strong wills to take care of their own needs. They can run and play, eat, have tantrums, and zoom through life ricocheting off of its experiences. They gradually grow and learn to live with themselves, others, and society's demands. As they mature, they gently learn of mortality and other hard lessons of living.

Children with diabetes do not have the leisure of gentle learning. They are confronted very quickly with death and the many ugly ways that a person can rush to it. They are told graphically of the disease's complications. Sometimes, they see them. Blindness, renal failure, and circulatory decay are not fairy tales. They are rushed into a life demanding at best careful discipline and at worst rigid control. They are told what to eat or not to eat, when and how to exercise, how many and what kind of shots to take, and how to regulate almost every other facet of their lives. They can feel like prisoners of a body that has betrayed them by having diabetes. They experience fear, anger, despair, and desperation in proportions well beyond those usually associated with being a child. They are forced in many way to be adults before their time.

The parents of children with diabetes do not enjoy a trouble-free emotional terrain. They frequently suffer with guilt because their child (or children) has a disease often considered hereditary. They may feel that they somehow passed the diabetes onto their child. They would prefer to endure the pain, uncertainty, and rigidity rather than have the child have to go through with it. If they cannot assume the disease, they want to make it up to him or her. Such thoughts as "Since he has diabetes, I won't give him a hard time about that" or "She's talking back to me because her sugar must be low" can interfere with the usual parenting process. The parent is torn between making it up to the child and being sure that the child assumes the responsibilities of becoming a mature adult.

Other times the children with diabetes can receive all of the parents' attention. Even if there are no other children to feel neglected, the one with the disease can be treated too delicately. Because so much can go awry, parents tend to hover. They help so much that they can be managing the child's disease. They can become overzealous excuse makers or policemen. They can become buffers between the child with diabetes and the realities of the day-to-day world. The child with diabetes can end up depending entirely upon the parents for everything.

The understandable—if not excessive—attention paid to the child with diabetes can set up the child as someone different or special. The disease can become the kid's primary claim to fame. Sometimes some children use the disease as an unfortunate means for soliciting attention: extremely high sugars, very low sugars, overdosages of insulin, forgotten medication, and ignored exercise programs are common strategies.

Extraordinary attention can result in social difficulties. In the family, the children without diabetes may resent what they perceive to be unequal treatment. Lesser causes have ended up in severe sibling rivalries and divided families. Outside the family, the child may feel like an outsider because he or she has diabetes. While at home it may be great to be different or special, but in school and social settings feeling different somehow can be a curse to be avoided at all cost (such as totally ignoring identification jewelry). Trying to be "normal" becomes a destructive, futile quest.

Thinking about the complexities of being a parent could puzzle the brightest and the best. Considering the added difficulties inherent in being the parent of someone who has diabetes could paralyze the stout-hearted.

But the task is too important. Few need be reminded of the value of being effective parents to youngsters. But effective parents are even more important to children with diabetes. While being a parent to a child who has diabetes is tough, demanding, and complicated, effective parenting is essential for the wellness of the child as a person as well as a person with diabetes.

Effective parents—whether for children with or without diabetes—serve best when they help their offspring become independent, self-sufficient people. Parents can contribute to their effectiveness by considering the complex emotional landscapes of being a parent, a child, and a person with diabetes. They can contribute further by insisting upon the child's participation in his or her own life. When a child senses that he or she can function efficiently and confidently on his or her own, the child will be equipped for living life. While overprotecting a child may cultivate self-pity, insecurity, and timidity, the insistence upon the assumption of responsibility helps the child believe that life is to be lived rather than run from, that problems can be solved, and that the difficulties or disorders need not prevent a person from having a full and rich life.

Rather than doing for the children, the parent can help them learn to do for themselves. Watching the diet, adjusting the insulin, choosing the exercise program, and dealing directly with the health-care professionals represent a few of the things children with diabetes can learn to do for themselves. When they learn such crucial things and assume responsibility for them, they are free to strive for wellness on their own, to savor the success of their own therapeutic programs, and to take on responsibilities beyond handling diabetes.

The child can be free, the parent can be free, and the relationship between parent and child can be based on things other than diabetes. Not only will the children be on a path of wellness regarding their diabetes, but also they can look to a positive approach to living in general. The parent will have a partner in the risky business of parenting.

Waiting for a Cure

FREQUENTLY, WHEN TALKING about diabetes, those of us with diabetes try to include some discussion of the research being conducted which seeks a cure or "painless" miracle treatments for our disease.

Some of us focus on historical accounts of the seemingly rapid improvements in the treatments of diabetes and point to such remarkable "progress" as a clear indication of things to come. Others are excited about the potential of future developments such as non-pricking blood glucose monitoring, suppository insulin, insulin infusers, closed-loop pumps, the artificial pancreas, organ transplants, and vaccines.

Such topics, it seems to me, are good to include in our discussions of diabetes. One reason might be our desire to inform each other of the progress being made in diabetes research. It helps us all be knowledgeable about current developments. Perhaps another reason for looking to the future is that it gives us hope. When I talk about diabetes, I agree it's important to include hope. Sure, the history of diabetes and its treatments, the nature and the symptoms of the disease, the ways of treating it, and the possible complications involved in the disease should be covered in responsible discussions. But to focus solely on medical history, medical treatments, or personal "war" stories can make for dull or boring or depressing conversation. Hope offers an attractive alternative.

However, while I understand the need for hope, I am concerned about how helpful an overemphasis on such promises for the future can be. To me, taking too much stock in the promise or the possibilities of future cures or miraculous treatments for diabetes does not make much sense. In fact, such hope, it seems to me, can be very dangerous.

A person waiting for a cure or for the development of miraculous treatments for diabetes (or the complications developing from it) reminds me of what many people today are doing about pollution and other threats to the environment. Despite the often-repeated warning about the dangers to our air, water, and ground, most people seem undisturbed and unwilling to do much to deal with the real threats to the quality of their lives.

Why? They are confident that science or God or some other agent will rush in and save them. They believe that a machine or a chemical or a miracle will be discovered or invented or created that will purify and save the air, the water, and the ground. Any day now, as so often before, they will be snatched from the abyss of pollution by some marvelous discovery or event. It is inconceivable to them that, unless they do something themselves, they will not be saved. They have confidence in our ingenuity, creativity, and intelligence. They are certain that we are the Chosen People. They derive hope from their absolute faith in progress. Because of this faith and resulting hope, they do not feel compelled to do much of anything about unbreathable air, undrinkable water, and the poisoned ground.

I hope they are right. If they aren't, the consequences of such misplaced faith and hope can be devastating.

Similarly, I don't think people with diabetes should place too much faith in the progress of medical research. To live with the hope that a cure or miraculous treatment will be discovered is only human and understandable. (I wish that the cure had been found yesterday.) But to count on such progress and therefore to become passive in dealing with diabetes on a day-to-day basis seems foolish. As with those who are counting on an environmental miracle, those waiting for a vaccine or a pancreas transplant had better be right. If they aren't, the disappointment can be devastating.

Waiting for a cure takes more faith than I can muster. I do not have the temperament that would allow me to sit back with a passive confidence that it will all work out. The odds for such a gamble seem much too long for me.

Perhaps I am a pessimist, but I am unwilling to take the risk that the cure or miracle treatment would be one day too late. The cost of being wrong is too high. I prefer to work with the here and now. I would rather wrestle with the problems directly than surrender my fate to the promise of progress. I don't have the fortitude it would take to let the quality of my life decline until progress swoops in and saves me. Living with diabetes in passive anticipation of a cure or a miracle treatment would be like breathing foul air, drinking contaminated water, and tilling poisoned soil with the hope that things would be better. I prefer to frolic as much as possible while actively battling the diabetes.

I never was much good at waiting. I am even worse when the odds are long.

A Physician's Response to "Waiting for a Cure" by Marvin C. Mengel, M.D.

THE PROMISED LAND was anticipated, predicted, and even guaranteed, and a band of weary nomads finally was able to enter. However, several things about the Promised Land are important to remember. First, while waiting to enter, a whole generation of people had died in the desert. Second, upon entering, the surviving nomads were sent the message to "be strong and courageous." Rather than "sit back and enjoy," the message was "be prepared to work." Entering the Promised Land provides the opportunity, but pain, heartaches, and difficulties had to be endured before the benefits were to be realized.

I sense a great similarity between the weary nomads and the health-care professionals and patients who are looking to the Promised Land of a cure for diabetes. Many believe today as if someday the doors will open, we can get on the elevator, and we will ride untroubled to the ultimate plane of diabetes treatment.

I hope, and expect, that someday there will be a cure. However, we all need to remember a few important points. First, this generation may not be around to see a cure or to benefit from it. Second, a cure will not reverse damage already done to the body. The cure probably will be one that will reverse the intolerance of carbohydrates. It will allow an individual to have functioning pancreatic tissue to keep blood sugar normal. The way it will be a cure is that it will, without effort on anyone's part, allow an individual to maintain a normal blood sugar. But, when the cure is found, the blind will not then see, the lame will not then walk, and the dead will not then live. At best, kidney disease, eye disease, circulatory disease, and nervous system disorders may be halted in their intrusion. For many people, though, the permanent damage already will have been done. For others, the damage may be so extensive that its effects will continue to do damage, even with consistently normal blood sugars after the cure. Studies have shown that kidney failure and eye disease reach a certain point at which, even with newly instituted ideal control, deterioration continues.

Thus, for the generation of people who presently have diabetes, the day of the cure may hold more frustration than hope. Rather than being free of the disease, they may be lamenting: "If only I had taken better care of myself" or "Now that my blood sugars can stay normal, if only I didn't have such and such a complication."

The idea of a cure, therefore, requires re-examination. Rather than an instant, easy paradise, it should be thought of in terms of a Promised Land which will require strength, courage, and work to reach.

For those with Type II diabetes ("late onset" diabetes, when a person's insulin receptors are too few or malfunctioning), the cure is here. The Promised Land awaits. They need simply to open the door and enter. The desert beasts which keep them from the Land are the refrigerator, the convenience foods, the self-destructive need to overeat, and the refusal to exercise. To be cured, people with Type II diabetes have to have the strength and the courage to face down the desert beasts which have, in many cases, caused their disease and which will bring it to its tragic conclusion. By facing them down, they can get their blood sugar down to normal and thereby restore their pancreatic physiology back to normal. By doing these things, their glucose tolerance test can be normal, the cure can be obtained, and the gates to the Promised Land will be opened. Thus, without resorting to any miraculous drugs or any expensive concoctions or gadgets, people with Type II diabetes can be free. Certainly, the task is difficult, but the opportunity exists now.

People with Type I diabetes (insulin dependent), probably would kill for such an opportunity. They must wait for a discovery or a concoction or a gadget. However, the promise of a possible cure for Type I diabetes should be used as motivation to keep the best possible control now to prevent the occurrence of complications and thereby "keeping the finger in the dike" with the hope that someday soon the cure will come. By being "strong and courageous" before the Promised Land is to be entered, a person with Type I diabetes will be in better condition to reap benefits from the cure when it arrives.

What might carry those with Type I diabetes into the Promised Land? One possibility is the use of immunosuppressive drugs which are used when the disease first starts before the beta cells have been completely destroyed. It seems that Imursan and Cyclosoporin do hold some hope in preventing the progression of the disease and even allowing its reversal. Unfortunately, the drugs' side effects may be worse than the disease. Furthermore, this type of cure holds no promise for those people who already have Type I diabetes. It simply spares beta cells still alive; it does not renew them.

For those whose diabetes is in full force, other approaches will have to be used. One is not really a cure but a mechanical device—a close loop artificial pancreas. Another is to find a way to provide new beta cells—by transplanting a pancreas or implanting new individual beta cells—which would recognize blood sugar levels, produce insulin, and release it as needed.

Though there are some signs of hope on the horizon of the Promised Land, only time will tell whether these approaches will blossom into the cure or whether they simply will give us more information on which another generation of researchers will build. But we will need to be "strong and courageous." When the device or devices or techniques to cure diabetes are developed, there will need to be much experimentation. There will be failures. There will be many disappointments. For example, with beta cell implants, they may work awhile, and then perhaps in a few years the body may destroy them. The disease will start all over again. On the other hand, new complications that we are not aware of may develop from the cures themselves. Plus, the cure may not be total or may not be instant; years of study will be required and close follow-ups will have to be conducted before the cure is declared indeed a cure—one that works without problems.

In short, physicians and patients alike need to be "strong and courageous." The often-expressed hope for a cure for diabetes is a desire to escape from the present realities. One cannot blame anyone for wanting to escape diabetes. But saying it will not get it done. People with Type II diabetes will have to face down the desert beasts by curtailing their eating and by exercising. People with Type I diabetes are going to have to do the best they can with present-day treatments: they will be in the best condition to be candidates for the cures that will become available and to be able to take advantage of what they have to offer. They also will be the ones chosen as the first subjects to try the cures out.

But the reality is that the cure will not wash away the devastation wrought by the disease over the years. It will provide only the maintenance of blood sugars without personal intervention. The cure can only alleviate the necessity for personal involvement. The irony then is that even now we have the ability to maintain fairly normal blood sugar levels with maximum personal involvement. Now we are working on the utilization of insulin pumps and the possible use of intraperitoneal insulin which will improve the levels of control currently being experienced.

So, the "cure" of diabetes, to a certain degree, exists now for Type I and Type II diabetes. Therefore, the goal should be to maximize present therapy rather than to take it easy, relax, and wait for future cures and benefits. We need to remember that the Promised Land came only after much sacrifice, and it demanded strength, courage, and hard work.

PART III

Feelings

Feelings

I MADE A BIG MISTAKE decades ago and compounded that mistake for decades. I didn't allow myself to admit to any feelings about my having diabetes. I didn't allow myself to consider what or how I felt about the disease. I hadn't cried, screamed, or even been angry about the disease. For years after the diagnosis when I was nine years old, I behaved "well." I was cool, calm, and philosophical about having diabetes.

I was stupid. It is dumb to deny having feelings about a disease that does so much to screw up one's life.

For decades I pretended to be very "adult" about the whole thing. For years I resigned myself quietly to the pains associated with having diabetes.

"Yes, isn't it just wonderful that they have insulin to virtually cure the disease."

"Certainly, all one has to do is to follow doctor's orders, watch that diet, exercise regularly, and keep track of several hundred other details and I can lead just as normal a life as anyone."

"They are doing wonders with lasers in treating the eye problems of those with diabetes."

"Indeed, I am truly lucky to have a disease that isn't as serious as cancer."

"Perhaps some chance exists that someone with diabetes can have problems sexually and may have children with diabetes, but the odds seem to be improving."

"Yes, it is a stroke of luck having diabetes so I wasn't drafted and didn't have to go to war."

"No, it doesn't bother me that you are gorging yourself on Halloween candy in front of me."

"Sure, I'm sure, Coach—I'm allowed to go out for football. There's no reason I can't play."

"Gee, I'm sorry, Brucie. I can't stay overnight at your house on account of all this stuff I have to do."

"Mom, why can't I stay home with Holly and Jimmy when you go to visit Dad in the hospital?"

"What do you mean, Dad, that I'll never lead a normal life?"

Such recollections point out to me that diabetes has always seemed to be the barrier between me and perfect happiness. I have always felt different and not in a good way. I hate diabetes. But I never allowed myself to admit that openly. I refused to acknowledge any resentment and therefore wouldn't permit such feelings as anger, fear, sadness, or hopelessness.

I bottled everything up. Submerged and unexamined, each unexpressed feeling itself became, in turn, a barrier to any semblance of peace or happiness for me. By pretending that such feelings did not exist, I pretended that everything was okay. I pretended to be properly resigned to having diabetes. Unfortunately, it was not authentic and inhibited genuine peace with myself and my diabetes.

So dumb.

So here goes: I hate diabetes! I hate being "diabetic." I don't want to be known as a "diabetic." I resent having to watch my diet. I feel hemmed in by a schedule that I find unyielding. I am weary of every meal and every action requiring a major set of decisions of how much, when, and why.

I am fed up with threats. I am sick and tired of waiting for the complications to set in. I cringe just thinking about what the next health-care provider will warn me about. I am sick of trying to figure out how much time I might have left. I am frustrated by the imprecisions of a medical science that cannot tell me what an ice cream cone, an insulin reaction, or a missed exercise period will cost me.

A life filled with unanswered questions nauseates me. Why was I picked out to have diabetes? What did I do to deserve such a life? Why will all those idiots who eat themselves into rotundness, refuse to exercise, and smoke like chimneys outlive me? Why in heaven's name can't medical research guarantee that doing such-and-such will prolong my life? When will they find a cure?

I refuse to be grateful "that it isn't worse." I am irritated by people who assure me that I can be "normal" or pity me because I will "never lead a full life." I am fed up with people watching me. I want my life back! I miss a lot of things such as apple pie, getting drunk, doing wild and crazy things to excess, and planning for retirement.

I am tired of having diabetes. I am worn out with being mature, with trying to be brave, with pressing on regardless, and with concealing my base emotions. I want to let out my primal feelings and not feel guilty or embarrassed, I want to smash something or scream out loud or cry myself to exhaustion.

I *am* going to let go! I *am* going to let myself feel! I *am* going to feel better!

Arrgh! #*&%$#!!!

I Am Not a Diabetic

I AM NOT A DIABETIC.

I will not be identified as a diabetic.

I will not be known as a diabetic.

I will not be reduced to a simple label.

I will not become a mere carrier or representative of a disease.

I will not have how I behave, feel, or think explained or dismissed because I happen to have diabetes.

People with diabetes are people trying to live in the twentieth century with shared hopes, fears, needs, and aspirations. Like all people, we share one attribute: each of us is an individual—a person with a unique combination of characteristics.

I am not a diabetic.

I am a person who has lived for forty-five years. During that period of time, I have been raised by my parents, gone to school for twenty years in eighteen different places, lived while four decades of history unfolded, married, fathered two boys, and done thousands of things in my own individual sequence and in my own individual way.

I am a unique product of those experiences.

I am not a Southerner or Northerner or any other geographical name place. I have lived in more than twenty places between Canada and Texas. I was born in Flushing, Long Island. I lived a few months in some places; nineteen years in one. My youth was spent primarily in the Northeast. I have lived in Orlando, Gainesville, and DeLand since coming to Florida in 1962. I don't have a southern accent.

Although I have done these things, I am not a biker or a tennis player or a fisherman or any other sportsman. Unlike star athletes who can become identified with their special event, I have played many sports and am not very good at any of them. I have been involved in organized baseball, football, wrestling, swimming, tennis, and basketball since I was nine. I also have enjoyed (suffered through) running, bicycling, fishing, racquetball, volleyball, hiking, bowling, and other unorganized activities. I have spent three weeks in the Rocky Mountains backpacking, five straight days in Las Vegas gambling, and hours on a golf course trying to hit a little white ball straight.

I am not a teacher, although I teach English. I have been known to dig septic tank drain fields, paint houses, build additions onto homes, go long-haul trucking, mow lawns, and program computers. I have worked for Midland Guardian Corporation and for AT&T as well as taught in a high school, a community college, a state university, and a private liberal arts college. I have done freelance writing and dismantled a television transmitter. I have not and will not accept the assertion that "those who can, do; those who can't, teach."

I am married and have two sons. But to me—and to them, I hope—I am more than a husband and a father. I'd like to think that we are also friends. Likewise, I have an existence beyond my emotional relationships with them and beyond my responsibilities to them. I am more than a protector and a provider. I do more than generate dirty clothes and dirty dishes, rules, and regulations. I am a person: weak as well as strong, afraid as well as brave, sensitive as well as hard, emotional as well as calculating.

To accept the traditional roles prescribed by such labels as "middle-aged," "Southerner," "jock," "teacher," "husband," or "father," is to reduce a complex me to a set of behavior patterns, social functions, and attitudes. Such labels often dictate how to act, think, feel, and live.

They can influence a person's view of his past, present, and future. Labels can seem to snatch the sense of free will from a person. They can control and trap and endanger the individual to whom they are assigned.

I am not a diabetic.

I will not allow the label to tell me who I am or what my life will be. I am a person who is going to live his life. I refuse the "diabetic" mantle—too many times it generates a group identity characterized by physical and emotional complications.

To accept the "diabetic" label allows others to see me only as a set of symptoms, a string of complications, and a certain dark future. I am more than what I can and cannot eat, more than the number of shots I take, more than the results of medical tests, and more than a bundle of impending problems. If I tolerate that label, doctors, fellow workers, acquaintances, and family members might assume that what I am doing, thinking, and feeling is simply the result of being "diabetic."

To accept the "diabetic" label may ensure my succumbing to things like nerve damage or despair. To refuse the "diabetic" label may help me to live a well-rounded physical and emotional life apart from the disease of diabetes. To focus on the things usually associated with the disease may contribute to their occurrence. I do not want that to happen. Even if they are to come, I refuse to spoil the life that I am living now by allowing the disease to overshadow all that I do, think, and feel.

Not accepting the "diabetic" label is one way for me to reject an over-simplified vision of me, to try to get others to treat me as an individual, and to resist my surrendering to the disease.

I am not a disease.

I am not a "diabetic."

I am unique.

I am an individual.

I am a person.

I am Mike Raymond.

Denial: Dealing with Death, Diabetes, and Other Inconveniences

Most people know intellectually that they will die. But they usually live their lives quite freely. In fact, they often carry on their pursuits of happiness in ways which seem to disregard the inherent dangers to their physical well-being. Some drive as if the car were a Sherman tank. They jaywalk with abandon. Others smoke cigarettes and cigars and drink to excess. Many gorge themselves on juicy red meats, fried foods, chocolate ice cream, and fast food delicacies. Few exercise regularly. When they do decide to break a sweat, they do not check with their doctor, do not warm up, and overexert.

Most people pursue the American Dream relentlessly. They work long, stressful hours. They work with people they dislike and in conditions that threaten their physical and emotional health. They often work more than one job. They frequently try to handle the multiple responsibilities of a career, a family, and a continuing education with the time, energy, and drive sufficient for only one set of responsibilities.

They don't play much differently. They play very hard and usually overdo it. In fact, they work at play. Leisure frequently is as hazardous as their deplorable eating habits and their stressful working routines. By the thousands, people have taken up sky diving, mountain climbing, ballooning, snow skiing, hunting, and motorcycle racing. They head into wilderness, dive into caves, and fly into the horizon without a second thought.

Whether just living day-to-day, working, or playing, people act as if they are indestructible. They behave as if they have a guarantee that their bodies will be immune to wear and tear, accidents, and/or disasters. They assume that everything which can go wrong will strike the other person. They know better. They know they are vulnerable to fate, chance, and desperate men. Intellectually, they know they will die, but emotionally they refuse to accept such an understanding. They deny they are mortal.

Some would argue that denial is hiding: maladaptive and unrealistic. I cannot agree. Denial permits us to live fully. For me, denial allows people to live freely, happily, foolishly, relentlessly, hazardously, and spontaneously. Without the denial of their mortality, many people would be unable to participate in the ordinary and extraordinary events of life. They would be unable to perform in the various arenas of daily existence. The fears that what they eat or what they do or what accident could happen would endanger their fragile existences certainly could paralyze them. Without the ability to block out the awareness of the human vulnerability, few could live full, productive lives—and fewer could be happy.

It is this same sort of denial that I have used and still use in order to live with my diabetes.

I have, in fact, practiced two forms of denial. One I will continue to practice; the other I would like to abandon.

The form of denial I follow but would like to abandon is "full-time" denial. Soon after the diagnosis of my diabetes and after my parents grew exhausted from their constant vigilance, I refused to admit that I had the disease. I refused to tell anyone about the diabetes; I made no concessions in behavior or diet. I joined the herd in pre-adolescent, adolescent, and post-adolescent behavior. Meals were frequently irregular and catch-as-catch-can. In fact, I used extreme behavior just to prove to myself and others that I really did not have diabetes. Strenuous sports and killer schedules including school, sports, and part-time jobs became obsessions. I was going to do it all.

As soon as I could practice "full-time" denial without someone jumping down my throat, the urine testing tablets, the gram food scales, the diet plans, the fasting blood sugars, and the regular doctor visits disappeared from my life. I hid my clinical diabetes manual as if its disappearance was linked to the presence or absence of my diabetes.

Of course, even then I knew that the "full-time" denial was as foolish a strategy as was hiding the diabetes manual. It wasn't foolish just because it wouldn't prevent all of those complications that the doctors had promised me. It was foolish because it didn't really allow me to escape the disease. As I took my one injection per day—a dosage and mixture of insulins unchanged for 28 years—I knew that I wasn't fooling myself with the full-time denial. No matter what strategies I employed, I couldn't relieve myself of the incredible anxieties that had been visited upon me with the original diagnosis of diabetes and my first stay in the hospital. As I skipped each old-fashioned urine test or regular doctor appointment, ignored every diet or parental admonition, and didn't take care of my feet or teeth, it was never far from my mind that I would pay dearly. In fact, this feeble "full-time" denial only exaggerated the worst part of diabetes—the fear. The more I pretended that I didn't have diabetes the more afraid I became of what I was doing to myself. The heightened fear didn't move me to be a "good diabetic." It became part of a vicious cycle: denial leads to fear which leads to more denial which leads to more fear. "Full-time" denial wasn't really effective because it didn't accomplish my objective of getting diabetes out of my life. It just exchanged treating the symptoms of the disease for worrying about the disease. Each day was one of waiting for the ax to fall: eyes? toes? legs? kidneys? death? whatever? Impending doom dominated every waking moment—and turned some dreams into nightmares.

Sure, I called it "full-time" *denial*, but it wasn't. In reality, it was just full-time *worrying* and *waiting*. It didn't work.

Part-time denial, on the other hand, has been more useful. Part-time denial allows some freedom from the potentially paralyzing grip of diabetes. Essentially, with this form of denial I forget that I have the disease between injections and meals. Now this is no easy task: I take injections and eat four times a day! But I forget I do. And it works.

When I get up in the morning, I do the glucose self-monitoring, adjust my insulin, take my various medications, and eat breakfast. When I get up from the breakfast table, I don't have diabetes. I charge off to work focusing only on the challenges, the adventures, and the sloughs of despair that everyone faces each day.

When the lunch hour arrives, I have diabetes again—for about five minutes. I close my office door, whip out my glucose monitoring and insulin apparatus, and do the necessary business. As I open my door and stroll off to lunch, I leave the diabetes in my desk drawer. This is the pattern for dinner and for the bedtime snack.

Once the business is done I deny that I have diabetes. I refuse to let it dominate my thinking, my feelings, my perceptions of myself, or my plans.

For the four or five hours between injections, I pretend I am free. I deny that I have diabetes. I insist that I am healthy. I am adamant that I can do whatever anyone else can do. I am certain that I have as much of a future as anyone. My portion of the American Dream is as guaranteed as anyone's. I will work hard and long to earn fame, fortune, and an occasional raise. I will play competitive sports until I am old and gray. I will need a retirement plan. I will bounce my grandchildren on both knees.

Given the oppressive evidence of the statistics and the hundreds of diabetes case histories, the part-time denial sounds as silly as hiding the diabetes manual. Nevertheless, it works for me. On the one hand, part-time denial permits me the freedom to go on about living my life. For all but about three hours a day I can revel in the immortality that those without diabetes assume is theirs. I then too can live freely, happily, foolishly, relentlessly, hazardously, and spontaneously. What good would it do for me to huddle in my house and lament the oppressive statistics and the case histories? I will not be defined by a disease or inhibited by it. If they are accurate and if I am to become another one of the statistics tomorrow, it makes sense to me to live as fully as I can today. Part-time denial doesn't allow diabetes to spoil the texture of life for me.

On the other hand, with part-time denial, I am not haunted with industrial-strength worrying and waiting. By admitting that I have diabetes three hours a day, I can monitor the blood sugars, adjust the insulin, and follow a diet. I believe that I am doing what is necessary and what is good for me. I am treating the diabetes. I am doing the best that I can do. As a result, I am not constantly haunted as I was when I practiced full-time denial. I am doing what is possible to prevent the horrors that have been promised me for so long. There is no sense worrying about them all the time. What good would it do? Part-time denial gives *me* the rest of the day; it isn't the disease's. This form of denial gives me the strength, the courage, the will to live, and the will to live positively.

Accepting Diabetes: The Bottom Line
by Marvin Mengel, M.D.

MANY PEOPLE WITH diabetes and those who treat them believe that the patient's acceptance of his or her chronic disease is crucial for the successful treatment of diabetes. Considerable effort can be used in conducting the patient's battle to gain acceptance and to discard denial. I am not certain how primary acceptance should be in the therapeutic alliance.

What is acceptance? What does it mean to accept the fact that one has a chronic disease? As a physician, I find it easier to suggest what happens when a person does not accept his or her diabetes. Sometimes, they have problems even using the word "diabetes." They will say, "My sugar is high and I need to take insulin, but I don't have diabetes." Clinically, physicians say that those patients who miss appointments, refuse to wear identification, and are "poorly cooperative" are defined as having difficulties accepting their disease. They "breach their therapy program." In contrast, patients who seem to accept their diabetes are those who resign themselves to the disease and do what is necessary to treat it. Oh, they may cry at first, get depressed, or fly into a rage, but soon after diagnosis they get down to work on treating the diabetes.

The refusal to get down to work—the refusal to accept the disease—represents to many patients and physicians a form of denial. They contend that denial is a part of having a chronic disease. In fact, some insist that it is a crucial stage that has to be worked through by the patient before he or she is able to get down to work. Others refuse to grant that denial is a stage: they believe that it can be an important part of the patient's on-going coping mechanism. They contend that denial serves the patient as much as diet or exercise or insulin or medication. By using denial, the patient then can go about living.

Certainly, the patient's acceptance of diabetes is ideal. Perhaps denial can prove useful for those who cannot achieve acceptance. But, for me as a physician, the bottom line is control. Whatever degree of acceptance or denial there is, it should not interfere with the medical care of the disease.

No matter how little acceptance or how much denial, people who learn they have diabetes must learn the essential steps for self-care. If they have Type I diabetes, they should monitor their blood glucose levels, take their insulin, follow their diet, exercise regularly, and maintain medical follow-ups. The bottom line is the control of blood sugar levels: the necessity of maintaining normal blood sugars and normal hemoglobin A1C tests.

I can appreciate the problems of wrestling with the acceptance or denial of the chronic disease, but, as a physician, I am more concerned with the normalization of glucose for the prevention of chronic complications. Given the state of the art of diabetes care, we of the medical community assume that there is a direct correlation between control and the development of complications. While good control may or may not prevent the development of complications, most physicians agree, at worst, it will delay their development. The medical care of the disease has to be primary because of the ravages done to the body if the diabetes is not treated. Compared to heart disease, kidney failure, neuropathy, and blindness, the problems with acceptance and denial are relative luxuries. The bottom line has to be control.

What if people with diabetes find that they are human? What if they slip up? If blood sugar control is somewhat less than ideal? What if their behavior contributes to this lack of healthy control? Physicians have to ask what the problem might be. We must consider the possible problems. Have the patients not truly learned the primary goal for treatment? Have they not really learned how to attain the goal of control? Or is it that they have not intellectually agreed that control is the goal? Perhaps they agree intellectually, but for some human reason cannot live up to the standards.

The physician's responsibility is to determine if more office visits are necessary, if more information should be provided, or if counseling is called for. The patient's responsibility is to participate in the search to identify the problem or problems which prevent good control and to take advantage of the solutions offered. The patient must recognize that poor blood sugars and hemoglobin A1C results are destructive and a threat to longevity. Physicians and patients must pursue all available resources for attaining glucose normalization.

This is when, it seems to me, that working on acceptance should enter into the therapeutic alliance. When patients work to correct high sugars or a poor hemoglobin A1C, they are working on acceptance. They must be helped to see that the bottom line is control and the health that comes with it. By getting the patient to work first on control, the physician has in turn gotten the patient to accept to some degree his or her diabetes.

Acceptance is important. Investigating the inner workings of one's psyche is worthwhile. By working with a counselor, a support group, a friend, or a physician who will listen, people with diabetes can achieve significant progress in self-understanding, acceptance, and therefore a better handle on their chronic disease. But control is more important. It should be the first goal. Whether patients intellectually or emotionally accept their diabetes is not as crucial as their taking the steps to achieve healthy glucose levels. The bottom line is long-time control. The issue of acceptance or denial is determined by what the person will do to achieve the bottom line.

After the Honeymoon

THE RAYMOND CLAN rushed home from the diabetes care unit armed with new insulins, a new diet, and a blue binder full of new information. We bubbled with unbridled enthusiasm. The hospital's diabetes specialist had convinced us to join them in a "team" approach and had helped us build a program for wellness.

An 1800 calorie, high fiber diet? Hooray! Four glucose tests a day? Why not? Four shots a day? Sure!

Seven months went by. The glow disappeared.

I tried very hard to be good. I followed the diet, monitored my glucose, adjusted and took the shots.

But I missed juicy steaks, was tired of sore fingertips from pricking them for a drop of blood, and had not grown any fonder of needles. Day-in and day-out the tests, the decisions, the choices, the pain, the blood, the doctors' visits, and the expenses had worn down the glow Judy, Eric, Bryan, and I had shared when I had come home from the diabetes care unit.

But such inconveniences could have been better tolerated if my body had stopped betraying me. The sugars climbed and dove without apparent cause; no symptoms appeared to signal a reaction; the right eye hemorrhaged.

I tired of waiting for the next "event." I found myself depressed. I just didn't want to do what I knew I should have been doing.

What happened to the honeymoon?

What could I have done to rekindle the flames of that earlier zeal?

Had a cold beer? What about a Snickers bar? A whole cheesecake? Taken time off from doing the glucose monitoring? Retreated back into my old "I'm not diabetic" closet? Asked someone to repeat a familiar sermon about how important it is for me to monitor, to diet, and to regulate?

What should I have done?

Perhaps I could have checked into the unit for a transfusion of their dedication and enthusiasm. Maybe a telephone call to one of the unit's health providers who could have reconnected me to a realistic and humanistic attitude towards a disease that seems especially adept at shorting out my common sense? (The call would have been cheaper than a hospital stay!)

Maybe Buster was right—perhaps the time had come for me to seek out one of the support groups. Maybe some of the more than thirteen million people with diabetes out there had had the same experiences and would have been willing to share their feelings and suggestions for combatting the post-honeymoon despair.

The honeymoon was certainly over. I smacked right into the frequently grim discrepancies between my idealized expectations and the hard realities of living with (against?) diabetes.

What did I do?

I called up a friend, challenged him to a tennis match, adjusted my insulin, took my one good eye, and thrashed him soundly.

The Other Side of Progress
by Marvin C. Mengel, M.D.

Those at all familiar with diabetes know the basic history of diabetes mellitus. Described several thousand years ago, the disease had been rapidly fatal and remained so until well into the twentieth century. Then, with the discovery of the hormone insulin, hopes for a cure began to grow. Blood sugars were brought down; lives were saved.

Unfortunately, the excitement about having found a cure for diabetes soon dimmed. Patients continued to have problems controlling blood sugar levels and began to develop problems. As the patients lived longer, they developed new problems or complications from the stress that the disease puts on the body. Over the last 60 years, diabetes has become one of the leading causes of blindness, kidney failure, and amputation. People with diabetes have been very susceptible to heart attacks and strokes.

In the last five years or so, hopes for a new age in diabetes care have developed again. Home glucose monitoring, new insulins, insulin pumps, and the hemoglobin A1C test (which indicates the level of control of glucose over two to three months) were among the advances which enhanced the treatment of the disease's symptoms. More importantly, evidence has begun to accumulate which indicates that keeping blood sugars in relatively normal range will decrease—if not prevent—the long-term complications which have plagued those living with diabetes. Now, more attention and more funding are being directed toward diabetes research. Dedicated people around the world are working hard to ensure that these new hopes do not dim.

Indeed, this progress seems remarkable. However, another side to this "progress" exists.

Consider, for example, what a patient said to me in anguish during an appointment in my office: "Sure, these things help. In fact, I really appreciate that, but they also make *my* failure more obvious."

With the progress in treatment techniques and the increased confidence by health-care professionals that the new systems can work, patients can feel a pressure that develops from there being opportunities "greater than ever before." What happens when the blood sugars don't come down although the person with diabetes is following his therapeutic regimen? When the hemoglobin A1C stays abnormal despite maximum effort? When even the numbers are "good" and the complications develop anyway? The patients feel like failures.

Patients and physicians need to remember the *fact* that people with diabetes are people first and unique people at that. As a physician, I am all too aware of the fact that endocrinology is frequently a mystery and that we have too, too much to learn. I need to remind myself to tell my patients that, while a treatment has been developed and seems to work with most people with diabetes, their particular system may be doing something different than what others have experienced. Medicine is a science, but I need to remind them that it is at best an imperfect one. Perhaps then we— the physicians and the patients—can overcome that sense of failure and press on for more progress.

Another by-product of "progress" has been the increased talk about people with diabetes being able now to lead a "truly normal life." In reality, people with diabetes are able to do "normal" activities, but their lives are far from normal. Talk about a "truly normal life" provides a mixed message. The results of this mixed message can be dangerous. On one hand, it suggests that there is nothing wrong. It indicates that diabetes is no excuse for not fulfilling the responsibilities of work, personal relationships, and community service. Furthermore, it is no excuse for poor performance. Many tend to forget that having a chronic disease is an additional responsibility that requires time, energy, opportunity, and money. It takes most of us without diabetes all the time we have—and more than we have—to do our work, to hold a job, to be a spouse, to be a parent, to be a friend, to be socially responsible, and to get through each day. People with diabetes not only have these same responsibilities, but also must invest extra resources to manage their disease. Ignoring the realities of these added responsibilities and not warning the patient with diabetes about them can set a person up for frustration ("Why can't I do it all? Everyone else seems to.") and an intensified loathing of the diabetes ("If I didn't have diabetes, I wouldn't be so messed up!"), which can result in treatment being ignored.

On the other hand, the talk of leading a "truly normal life" that has come from progress sends an implied message that is very dangerous to the person with the disease. The zesty emphasis on "normal" encourages the patient to ignore the diabetes. "Be normal" countermands the efforts to get people with diabetes to do the things essential for managing a chronic disease. How can people feel "normal" when they have to test their own blood, follow special diets, give themselves injections, or test their urine for ketones? Diabetes is a disease that demands discipline, and it is a discipline that few people without a chronic disease have to practice. To promise that they can be like everyone else is to set up frustration—if not to give license for ignoring the disease. As a physician, I want to give my patients something to hang onto, something that gives them an incentive to take advantage of the new research and treatments, but I have to be careful about promising a "truly normal life."

The focus of care, then, must not be on the progress and the new developments in diabetes treatment. It should be on the person. The specifics of treatment—and the application of new "tools"—must be individualized so that, as much as possible, the treatment fits the patient rather than the reverse.

As a physician, I try to bridle my enthusiasm for the progress inherent in the new tools, the new techniques, and the new data. There have been some dramatic improvements in diabetes treatment. However, I have seen too many people who have not enjoyed the benefits of such progress. I am too conscious that all the methods in the world are useless unless the people who are patients use them and use them gladly. The proper application of the new developments demands that we remember that we are treating *people* who have a disease, and not a *disease* that happens to occur in people.

When that happens, then I will take full pleasure in the progress in diabetes care, and I will have greater confidence that the hope will not dim.

Crunching Numbers

Do you recall the conversation the last time two or more people with diabetes or a patient with diabetes and a doctor got together? Did it go something like the following?

"How long have you had it?"

"About 36 years."

"Are you on insulin?"

"Four shots a day."

"How much insulin do you take?"

"Usually 10 to 14 in the morning, 2 to 6 at lunch, 6 to 12 at dinner, and about 2 and 10 at night."

"How have your sugars been running lately?"

"Anywhere from 400 to 40. I try to keep it around or below 180, but sometimes the morning sugars run about 240 to 400, and, of course, I have gone higher than 400 when I binge."

"What was your last HA1C?"

"Eleven-point-five."

"Do you have any problem with insulin reactions?"

"Sometimes about 2 to 4 a week, usually 3 hours after my morning injection."

"What is your calorie count?"

"Eighteen-hundred calories."

"What sort of diet are you on?"

"A typical dinner is 2 to 3 ounces of meat, 1½ cups of vegetables, 1 small potato, 2 slices of bread, and 1 small piece of fruit."

"Do you ever go off your diet?"

"About 3 times a month I go crazy. I eat 4 candy bars at one time or eat about 6 or 7 pieces of 3-inch pizza."

"How much do you weigh?"

"About 174 pounds."

"Is that a change?"

"I've lost about 5 pounds."

"Have you had any complications?"

"I have had 3 laser treatments on my right eye."

"What else?"

"I've had 2 hemorrhages in that eye due to the 2 laser treatments."

"Anything else?"

"Thirteen years ago I had 4 by-passes done on my heart; seven years ago, 3 more by-passes."

Numbers seem to dominate the treatment of diabetes. As a result, the numbers dominate the lives of people with diabetes—whether it is their conversations or the emotional terrain upon which they live with themselves and with those close to them.

Numbers are the tools for treating the disease. They have become a code or symbolic language for those in-the-know about diabetes. They indicate the "state" of the control: "good," "bad," or "crazy." They divide up the day; they mark when to eat and how much to eat; they tell how many times the person with diabetes takes injections. The numbers serve as historians who tell what has been going on and as fortune tellers who forecast the probable future (or non-future) for the person with the disease.

As well as the events of the day, numbers also tend to wield powerful control over the emotional lives of those with diabetes and those close to them. Families who hover and cower each morning as the resident patient does his or her glucose monitoring are common. Woe to them all if the strip darkens past the color combinations that denotes 180! Perfectly beautiful mornings and happy moods can be transformed in those three short minutes into a dark and stormy day of despair. The face of the person with diabetes darkens into rage in direct proportion to the colors on the strip. The family tiptoes around the house.

Furthermore, glucose testing is not the only touchy area connected with numbers. As the numbers on the syringe go up, so does the sense of guilt and despair by many people with diabetes. Although a large number have worked out a sliding scale (the amount of the insulin dosage changes according to the blood glucose level) after careful consultation with their doctors or diabetes specialists, many develop a 1929 Depression mindset about the amount of insulin their body requires. They act as if the amount of insulin available is restricted; the more they "spend" the more they are "wasting." Linked to this guilt is the sense that the more the insulin numbers go up the worse off they are and the darker their future. As the numbers increase, so does the despair.

Food even becomes part of the numbers-and-emotions landscape. Resentments easily develop as wheat thins are counted out, tablespoons of rice are measured carefully, and ounces of liquid are poured into graduated measuring cups. The accumulating numbers determine whether the person with diabetes is to be a "have" or "have-not" in each particular encounter with food. The rest of America lingers over the dessert tray as those with diabetes futilely refigure what they have coming to them. Everything edible seems to be in ounces rather than pounds, fractions rather than whole numbers, divided rather than multiplied. The relationship with food and with those who buy, prepare, or eat it is one of both love and hate. Frequently, the very reasons for eating, such as nutrition or pleasure, are lost or overshadowed by the battle over numbers: calories, amounts, sizes.

With the despair over the amount of insulin taken, the number of times insulin is taken, and the number of calories eaten (or not eaten) comes another set of numbers to darken the picture— number of years gone and of years left. While few talk of these numbers, even fewer would deny privately that such counting is frequently on their mind. "What will this high sugar cost me? How much time does this binge cost? How many years do I have left? When will the complications set in? Will I see my children finish high school?"

Not many would argue that counting years gone and years left doesn't make much sense. But, in a disease that depends so heavily on numbers, what else could be expected? Numbers lead to numbers; numbers provide patients, doctors, and nurses something tangible to work on. With a disease without a cure and where treatment is tricky, numbers offer opportunities for clear-cut objectives and a seemingly tangible "enemy." With numbers, perfectibility seems attainable. They can be used to measure success. They can suggest that the patient, the doctor, and the nurses are "winning" against the disease. Unfortunately, they also can be used to document failure, to record human imperfectibility, to threaten the person with diabetes, and to place blame. Thus, they can show that the "diabetic" is "losing." The record of apparent "losses" becomes a path to despair, guilt, fear, and a sense of deprivation. Despair tends to breed further despair. In short, numbers can be an ally and/or enemy.

How does this happen? Numbers represent a curious paradox. On one hand, they suggest science, precision, and answers; on the other, they are a large part of a guessing game. How much insulin one should take connects to how much one eats and how much exercise has occurred or will occur. The incalculable factor of stress adds another dimension for guessing. Glucose monitoring, calories, insulin units, heart rate, and minutes on the clock should add up to an exact science. But what frequently happens defies any attempts at causal explanation. Juggling all the numbers with the care of a mother handling a newborn baby often results in the primordial scream, "What is going on?!" Quickly that question can turn to "What's the use?" which indicates more frustration than a search for information. In general in our culture, science promises order, causation, and answers; in the science of treating diabetes, no such promises can be made or kept.

But knowing this discrepancy rationally does not ensure its acceptance emotionally. People with diabetes—and some doctors and nurses—become obsessive-compulsive about numbers. The numbers become a goal rather than a means for treating diabetes. Much like students who have replaced education with earning grades, people with diabetes (and their doctors and nurses) can make the numbers more important than the quality of their lives. The human gets lost in the pursuit of data, directions, or report cards. When the imperfect science goes awry—as it will—and the numbers go wacky, the human who has diabetes is very susceptible to being crunched. The wacky numbers become the same thing as an announcement of failure and of loss—they result in despair, apathy, depression, guilt, and fear. That, of course, ensures more wacky numbers and the deepening spiral into denial and noncompliance.

The person with diabetes has been crunched by the numbers.

What can we do?

First of all, try to remember that diabetes treatment is at best an imprecise and imperfect science. Expectations for simple, direct, and absolute connections between one cause and one effect are unrealistic. Too many unknown factors influence the numbers. Try to see the numbers as part of a procedure for treating the symptoms of diabetes. The numbers are a way to prescribe and to evaluate a therapeutic system, not the therapy itself. Obtaining the perfect numbers does not mean that the disease is beaten. Suffering with less than perfect numbers should suggest that the recent procedures might need to be modified if the numbers continue to come up that way, not that you have been beaten by the disease.

This will allow you to try to keep the numbers in perspective. A set of discouraging numbers does not signal the end of the world. The numbers are a way to head off an extended period of high numbers that may have unsavory effects. But, a day of "excess" calories, of "bad" sugars, and of "high" insulin requirements does not necessarily endure the "loss" of so many years, of so many limbs, or of so many normal human qualities. The numbers—especially high ones—provide an opportunity to avoid such consequences. They make the therapeutic system adjustable, flexible, and therefore human. Rather than the enemy, they allow a way to know each person's unique disease, a way for controlling it, and therefore a sense of not being its powerless victim.

By keeping the numbers in perspective you can try to avoid an emotional involvement with them. They do not point fingers. High ones don't scream, "You're bad!" or "You're dead!" Low ones don't sing, "You'll live forever!" In fact, most doctors or nurses don't intend to use them to make accusations. People with diabetes themselves seem most responsible for this nasty emotional nightmare of tying self-worth to the numbers. Sure the numbers can reflect a binge or some other human error. But what's the use of reacting as if they're the mark of Cain? If we surrender to the anger or despair, we end up avoiding the "bad" news": we don't do the numbers; we abuse those around us; we ensure more "bad" numbers. In short, we ensure all the things we are afraid of the most are going to happen. Numbers are history, not the future. Use them as tools for building.

Try to remember that having diabetes doesn't cut one out of the human race. As humans, people with diabetes can only do the best they can possibly do. No one expects more than the best we can do. Why should we expect any more from ourselves? To make unrealistic or unreasonable demands upon ourselves and to become emotionally upset when we don't meet these demands is to allow the numbers to crunch us. The numbers should not own us; they should be working for us.

On the Mountain

WHILE IN THE NORTH Carolina mountains for a family vacation, I made an unpleasant discovery. I wasn't as free of my diabetes as I had thought.

We had been to the mountain camp twice before, once four years ago and then just two years ago. Those two experiences had been wonderful for us as a family. From staying in a rustic cabin with a magnificent view to taking part in a full schedule of activities, Judy, Eric, Bryan, and I had reveled in the vacation "on the mountain." It had been great: we'd come back for more! I had had diabetes on those two previous trips, but not the way I did on this last trip.

Right after the trip two years ago, I had checked into a diabetes care unit for a complete physical evaluation and re-education. By the time I had checked out of the hospital, I found myself committed to a new diet, doing glucose self-monitoring, and taking multiple injections of new insulins daily.

The changes seemed worthwhile. I felt that I was fighting back against the diabetes. The more careful control and the more industrious management relieved me of the feelings that I was a passive victim of the disease. The regimen—while requiring more time, more information, and more effort—seemed to free me from many anxieties and to lessen the pressure from the "awful waiting." It also served as a source of personal pride because of the discipline it required.

But this last trip to the mountain has made me rethink my perceptions of the new management system. I was made acutely aware of the cost in using this new regimen. I didn't feel as free on the mountain as I had the two previous adventures. I didn't like the feeling.

For one thing, the desired goal of carefully controlled management system—consistently lower blood sugars—became a threat.

During this last trip, with having to climb the mountain just to get to meals—to say nothing of the many daily activities—insulin reactions became a constant possibility. It is no easy task to adapt a delicately balanced therapeutic triangle of insulin injections, diet, and exercise when breathing itself has become exercise in the thinner mountain air. The insulin schedule that I had brought with me had taken nearly three years to work out in a flat Florida terrain and a relatively established routine.

Once in the mountains, I was suddenly launching myself into day trips, nature hikes, waterfront activities, and other adventures scheduled morning, noon, and night. Who could tell which activity was going to produce plummeting blood sugars?

For the first time in my life, I found myself hesitating to participate in the fun and games. I became reluctant to take part in what was described as the tamest of activities. A rock slide or a river waterfall was no place for an insulin reaction. Plan ahead? Sure. But how much does one reduce the insulin? Even with two years' experience with the new regimen, I didn't feel that I was equipped to handle the changes in so many of the variables. How much more should I eat? When you are uncertain what your planned adventure involves, such decisions are not easily made correctly. At best, it is a guessing game that could be disastrous if you guess incorrectly.

What about an unplanned adventure? Consider one morning that was planned for quiet reading and relaxing in the cabin.

"Come on," Judy invited. "Let's walk down the mountain to the waterfront."

"Sure," I agreed. I grabbed a Snickers bar as we headed for the half-mile trail down through the woods.

At the bottom of the mountain, a sign beckoned us to a 1.5-mile trail to a waterfalls. Why not? I clutched the Snickers bar and tried to calculate how much breakfast I had eaten, how much insulin I had taken, and what sort of exertion this walk-turned-hike would require. Off we went.

A mile or so later (who could tell as we zig-zagged back and forth down a mountain?), another sign confronted us. It pointed downward and promised an amethyst mine in 1.5 miles and Blue Lake in three miles. What happened to Abe's Creek Falls? The sign made no mention of our original destination, and the only visible trail was down toward the mine and the lake.

"The falls must be on the way down."

No such luck. After 3.5 miles of steep, rugged trail, we found ourselves at the amethyst mine. We had been hiking hard for more than 45 minutes. I was damp with sweat and knew all too well that those breakfast calories were long gone and that my morning insulin was about to peak.

I sat down and slowly chewed the Snickers bar. I rested and waited for the chocolate, the caramel, and the peanuts to begin to digest. I had serious doubts about having enough glucose to make it back up the rugged mountain terrain 3.5 more miles. In fact, I feared that the candy bar's emergency calories were being consumed to handle the symptoms resulting from the journey down the mountain. As we began to retrace our steps, I could not help muttering, "This was a mistake."

The adventure turned out okay. We were back in our cabin in about an hour, and I quickly compensated for the unexpected exercise by eating nearly everything in sight. But the trek back had been hard. I dared not think about what might have happened. What if we both hadn't been in shape and had had to dawdle our way back up the mountains? I would have never gotten back in time to eat that supplementary food in time. What if we had gotten lost again? What if I hadn't grabbed that Snickers bar on impulse before we left for that "one mile walk"?

Needless to say, the unexpected adventure shook my confidence. Plus, I began to wonder about careful control. In the days before I had adopted my new regimen, my usual sugar levels would have proved more than ample to handle the unexpected. I had serious doubts about my being able to handle anything that was not scheduled. I began to feel vulnerable and inadequate and did not enjoy these new sensations. Perhaps the old method was better.

After the experience of going to the mine by accident, day-long trips were no longer an option to me. Besides the threat of insulin reactions, trips which had to involve a meal were too complex. How does one use a glucose monitor while white-water rafting? Give insulin injections while tubing down a river? Even a long placid hike becomes a problem with having to test the blood sugar and adjust the dose and eat. First, the equipment has to be brought along. While carrying the monitor, the test strips, the syringe, the insulin, and the emergency snack represents no real physical burden, how does one gracefully whip this stuff out among a bunch of strangers who are anxious to make tracks down the mountain trails?

Second, the meals are usually not calculated to fit a diabetes regimen. How does one tell the guide that a peanut butter and jelly sandwich, potato chips, chocolate chip cookies, and trail mix are not the meal of choice? What about being sure to be back to the base camp for the next snack or meal or injection? Sometimes it just doesn't work out. I didn't have the strength of character to assert myself—to insist that we have to be back to camp on schedule. Finally, one just feels restricted. You have to monitor the blood sugar, alter the insulin doses, and time the meals or else be walking blind with your diabetes.

I soon found that I had no stomach for such aggravation. It was easier to hide out in the cabin and to long for the good old days of one injection in the morning, high sugars, limitless reservoirs of energy and anonymity. The more I hid and the more I thought about the new regimen, the more I felt like a prisoner of diabetes.

But even hiding didn't disguise the costs and/or aggravations of the new regimen. In the old days of the previous vacations, before my new diet, I had enjoyed the quality and the bounty of an efficiently and intelligently run dining hall at the mountain. On the previous trips to the mountain, going to the dining hall three times a day was a joyous social and culinary occasion where even the most catholic tastes were usually fulfilled.

With this last trip to the mountain, meals were torture. The diet of my new regimen calls for complex carbohydrate combinations, vegetables, fruits, and high fiber. Red meats, cheeses, and eggs are to be avoided in order to eliminate concentrations of fat and cholesterol. My attempts to maintain a predominately vegetarian high-fiber diet were thwarted at nearly every meal. Eggs, bacon, sausage, pancakes, and sweet cakes dominated the breakfasts. Lunches were pork sloppy joes, hot dogs, beef soup, grilled cheese sandwiches, and peanut butter and jelly sandwiches. Dinner included pork chops, pot roast, beef stew, and creamed mystery meat. At first, eating was a challenge: how not to eat the meats, the eggs, and the cheeses and how to work up compensatory vegetable-and-bread combinations. But all too quickly I grew weary of the challenge and longed for the uninhibited "chow downs" of previous years on the mountain.

It wasn't just what I ate or didn't eat. Meals at the mountain were at 8:05 A.M., 12:35 P.M., and 6:35 P.M. So much for injections and meals every five hours! Adjusting to the breakfast and lunch schedule wasn't difficult and didn't take long, but the inter-val between lunch and dinner remained a hassle the entire week. Does one shoot up at the customary five hour interval and then tide oneself over at happy hour with beer, wine, and popcorn? I tried the popcorn-as-snack approach and paid with a reaction rebound. Once I even saved a snack from lunch, but in six hours it got pretty stale and I had some problems choking it down. Or does one wait until 6:00, get the discouragingly high blood sugar, and shoot up while everyone else is at the camp's social hour?

Decisions, decisions, decisions. Intellectually, I knew that this is the ordinary terrain of having diabetes and that even my usual routine at home on occasion involves such problems. But, on vaca-tion and at the mountain which provided such a glaring contrast, it suddenly seemed too much. I longed for the good old days of simplicity and freedom.

With each day the vacation became more and more of a reminder of that seemingly lost simplicity and freedom. What had been planned as a week for relaxation and rejuvenation first turned into a battle to remain compliant and to adhere to the therapeutic treatment plan. Then it darkened into grim depression. I became grumpy and angry. I wasn't fun to be around. As I became more and more aware of that trapped feeling, I became more and more in-wardly focused. Each day I hid out more and more. I spent most of my time weighing the merits of the new regimen in contrast to those of the old freedom and simplicity.

That preoccupation, of course, wasn't productive. Soon I felt even more trapped. I wanted the week to be over so that I could be back at home in the usual routines where I felt safer and comfort-able. This realization devastated me further. Too much of my life in the old days had been different, exciting, and had made no conces-sions to the diabetes. I had rarely been reluctant or hesitant to try anything. I had taken great pride in my avoidance of the 9-to-5 rat race and the sedentary routine which had eaten into the lives of many of those my own age or in the same social circumstances. I had been amused by those who had been at the mountain two and four years ago because they had gotten such a kick out of playing mountain men, Mr. Nature, and daring adventurers for one week a year. I had enjoyed those weeks because I had nothing to prove: I had been doing such things all year round for years. I had felt no urgency to prove myself. Now, all of a sudden, such pride seemed a farce. Apparently, in the last two years, I had slipped into a safe but stifling life of Walter Mitty. Yuck.

The fact that I had diabetes and that I had made an intelligent, rational decision to implement the new regimen in order to work for a longer life of some quality did not alleviate my despair. I felt like a wimp. I felt vulnerable and weak. The diabetes was jerking me around. The more I considered the safety of a structure and schedule and the benefits of the new regimen in treating the symptoms of my diabetes the more it drained me of my sense of vitality, strength, control, and yes—yes, as silly as it sounds—my manhood. I know better. I frequently admonish my sons and others about the silliness of measuring manhood or self-worth with such visceral standards. But the rationality provided no comfort. I lament the apparently lost freedom. I am sickened by the striking contrast between what I am now and what I used to be. I am embarrassed that I have been carrying on a charade for almost two years.

I wonder: Is the value of a new regimen worth the cost?

Out of Control

MY DIABETES IS OUT OF control. The blood sugars in the morning are running from 350 to over 400. I feel as if I had not had any sleep at all. I wake up in the morning exhausted. My legs ache, and my mouth is dry. I am very cranky. I have to take huge doses of insulin. I worry about what is going on.

By lunch time, the sugars are plummeting down to below 100. I feel weak, shaken, and anxious. I know that I must eat soon. I wonder what is going on. If the high sugars in the mornings are due to reactions, why does the sugar come down so rapidly?

The approach of supper time brings no assurances of what the glucose monitor will reveal. Sometimes the sugars are in the 110 to 180 range; other times they are in the 280 to 400+ range.

The bedtime sugars have rarely been a mystery lately: high and higher. It doesn't seem to matter what my activities have been that evening. If I play tennis, go to my office, wrestle with my sons, or just watch television, the sugars always seems to be in the stratosphere. I don't feel very perky: my body is lethargic, and I am very depressed.

Indeed, my diabetes is out of control. But I am depressed because I know why: *I* am out of control.

It isn't a simple mess. My being out of control comes in various complicated shapes. My lack of control becomes most evident with my insistence upon taking huge doses of insulin. I get disgusted with the high numbers and retaliate by taking so much insulin that I will be sure to see better numbers the next time. I usually go berserk with the insulin dosages during the morning and the bedtime injection.

My lack of control usually takes another form around lunch and dinner. As the blood sugar starts down and sinks below 90 and then 80, I foolishly refuse to acknowledge the symptoms which warn me of the approaching low sugar. I won't eat anything because I am afraid of another astronomical readout from the monitor. Of course, as the sugar goes down more and more, my abilities to rationally deal with the ensuing insulin reaction are by then too diminished to be helpful.

Then later, as the symptoms become too apparent to be ignored, my lack of control becomes extravagant. I start to eat. Then I keep eating. I don't stop eating. Rather than consuming just enough to halt the plummet to a dangerous insulin reaction, I turn into a frenzied pig—stuffing and eating without even tasting the uncounted calories.

After dinner—if the sugar is satisfactory or low—the eat-a-thon takes another extravagant shape. I start eating to prevent the frightening spiral of low sugars. A snack here, a little something there. The calorie intake moves into the four-digit range pretty quickly. I'm uncertain whether it's caused by a real fear of a feat of my imagination to justify the garbage disposal behavior. Who can tell when I'm out of control?

On the other hand, if the dinner sugar is high, the lack of control takes further bizarre turns. Sometimes I say to myself, "What the hell?" and cram the food in with dark perversity. On other occasions, after taking massive doses of insulin, I begin to "think" about how low I might go and start shoveling in the sinful food.

This description of my lack of control is much too orderly to be accurate. The chaos does not come in orderly paragraphs or a careful listing of separate types of disorder. The lack of control lashes out into my life like a violent story: ups and downs, fear and apathy, violence and passiveness, anger and disgust. It's all mixed up and confusing and irrational and savage and senseless. It's a mess that makes bigger messes.

But no matter how I tabulate the variations in losing control with diabetes or how I describe the impact of the chaos, it boils down to my failure to exercise discipline. I allow the disease to get out of hand, and then I let everything get away from me. I don't approach the high sugars as a problem to solve. I don't concentrate on the training I have had for diabetes management. I refuse to isolate the possible factors which may be contributing to the high sugar problem. I don't seek out the help of objective professionals who can offer advice. I allow my shame and embarrassment to prevent my admitting that the diabetes is out of control. I don't remain patient and calm. Rather than taking advantage of the disciplined reasoning emphasized through my education, I succumb emotionally to anger, fear, frustration, despair, and anguish. I slip all too quickly into an emotional spiral that contributes to a devastating lack of control.

When my diabetes is out of control, that usually means that I am out of control. When I am out of control, I have lost my mental and emotional discipline. I need to have discipline in order to live with my diabetes—just as any person needs discipline to live.

The Scapegoat

At the age of 32, I underwent open-heart surgery to have four arterial by-passes done. Nearly six years later at age 38 I underwent open-heart surgery again to have three more by-passes done.

The first adventure had been very traumatic. First of all, the need for the surgery had been a surprise. I was relatively young and—besides my diabetes—I was the apparent picture of health. Just before the chest pains had begun, I had been playing in tennis tournaments, had built a 30' by 12' addition onto my house, had been working full time, and had been conducting research in my spare time. I had never smoked, was not overweight, and was in pretty good shape. How could I have four blocked arteries?

Furthermore, the need for the surgery certainly had disrupted my family's lives. Our tentative plans for participating in the American Dream seem shattered. Just six months earlier, our second son Bryan had been born. My eldest child Eric was not yet three years old. I just had gotten some hope for job security at the university I had been teaching at for over six years. We had been living in our own home since Eric had been born.

Also, the need for the surgery had injected a large dose of fear into our lives. Certainly, the heart, its function, and that which affects it became central concerns in our lives. Every twitch of my body or article in the newspaper about heart disease sent me into a panic. But the fear wasn't restricted to the state of the heart. Throughout the process of the actual pre-operation work-ups, the operation, the recovery, and the recuperation, everyone commented, "You're so young! What caused this?...Oh, you have diabetes—that explains it." My once relatively silent adversary had become a viciously dangerous enemy. I had been fairly comfortable with the management of the diabetes: take care of it and forget it. No longer. It had been the culprit which had stolen up on my energetic body and had traumatized me and my family. The diabetes had reared its ugly head, and its threat was not only to my heart. Once silent and sneaky, it then seemed to stand like a raging, marauding barbarian waiting to ravage every part of my body. Diabetes became responsible for my winter sniffle, stubbed toe, jock itch, and balding head. Surely, the long promised complications had arrived.

The second bout with open-heart surgery made me mad. Judy, Eric, Bryan, and I had been working too too hard for such a recurrence so quickly. Exercise? Nearly every day! Diet? Friends and strangers admired my discipline. Medical care? Like clockwork! In fact, I had taken particular care to seek out the best diabetes care in the area. Relaxation? I had started taking vacations and had tried to limit moonlighting, course overloads, and teaching summer school. My pace certainly had been dramatically reduced compared to previous years. Judy had assumed all the "hassles" in our lives. We had been so very careful trying to do the "right" things to fight the heart disease and to manage the diabetes. Everyone commented enthusiastically on how well I looked and how healthy I seemed. I didn't fit the profile for "re-dos."

Then, boom!, a new set of scars that look like zippers!

Boy, was I angry! I had no trouble picking out a focus for the anguish, rage, and despair. It had to be that "damned diabetes." There was no beating that disease. Nothing was good enough. No matter what a person did, he paid. Diabetes means vicious surprises, fearful waitings, and dark disruptions. It had ruined my life, was ruining my life, and was robbing from me any semblance of hope. Damn, damn, damn diabetes!

I frequently found myself thinking, "If it weren't for diabetes, everything would be wonderful."

But that's not true—not for me, anyway. A more objective and rational examination of my circumstances reveals that diabetes is not the only villain for my heart disease. First, my father, who did not have diabetes, had a history of heart disease. He had, in fact, three massive heart attacks before the age of 38.

Second, even a cursory look at my life style since the beginning of time provides a classic instance of an obsessive-compulsive or Type-A personality. I had moved a million times, had gone to more than a dozen schools, and had been working since age nine. A shy and insecure person, I had suffered with having to leave friends and to make new ones and with having to adjust to a new environment every six months. The financial and emotional traumas caused by my father's medical problems and untimely death had generated even more pressure. Working my way through college, going to graduate school, and deciding upon teaching as a profession had not decreased the stress. Fighting for a tenure-track position on a university faculty when hired as a temporary instructor had forced me into long, tense hours of work after having graded seemingly endless piles of freshmen essays. Doing consulting work and moonlighting to supplement a beginning teacher's salary virtually had eliminated leisure and relaxation. My inherent insecurities seemed to have compounded the pressures.

Finally, when I considered my history of how I truly had dealt with my diabetes, I had to admit that I hadn't been that careful. In fact—time for true confession—I had been committing suicide by not just neglecting the disease, but actually conducting a seeming campaign to do everything I had been told not to do!

Sure, I can rant and rave about that damned diabetes. But, I must admit that I am probably using it as a scapegoat, something to blame for my heart disease. I know that historically diabetes has been correlated with the hardening of the arteries. However, I also must admit that family history and stress have been documented as major factors in causing heart disease. Also, the absence of control in the managing of the diabetes probably had compounded the damage connected with the heart disease. While the diabetes was an accessory, I shouldn't insist upon making it the major—if not only—villain in the crime. That, it seems to me, would be like blaming my father for my heart problems. I wouldn't be taking responsibility for my part in the whole process of clogging up my arteries, disrupting our lives, and injecting fear into daily events.

Furthermore, if I think about my use of diabetes as a scapegoat to blame for my heart disease, it occurs to me that I blame the disease for a lot of other things in my life.

It makes almost as much sense.

Certainly, if I did not have diabetes, I would not grow old. Those 19-year-olds on the other side of the tennis net would not be beating the tar out of me in tournaments. My hair would not be retreating at a gallop to the backside of my ears. That bulge oozing over my belt has to be from too many injections in the tummy. Without the wear and tear of the disease, I surely would be working and playing like I did in high school and college.

I am certain that either high sugars or low sugars are what makes me lose my temper, get impatient, or slip into depressions. Otherwise, I would be a model of human compassion, understanding, and equanimity. The disease is what makes me tired after working 18 hours straight or causes me to get the flu. Without the complex problems inherent with having diabetes, my whole life would be simple, pleasant, wonderful, and perfect.

Surely, it's that damned diabetes which has prevented me from being an ideal husband, a better father, a tennis champion, a world-known scholar, a best-selling novelist, and a middle linebacker for the Chicago Bears. I'd certainly be better looking too...and richer...and driving a red sports car...and out of debt.

I wonder what I would have done with the disappointments in my life if I did not have diabetes?

Feeling Good

Have you ever had "one of those decades"? You know, a period where everything seems to come apart or to fall apart or to go wrong for what seems like ten years in a row.

I have been through "one of those decades."

In December 1978, I underwent open-heart, by-pass surgery. At 32, I had a new set of plumbing installed: four coronary by-passes. I had spent three years trying to convince a series of doctors that I was experiencing severe chest pain. My "indigestion" was operated on over the Christmas holidays.

Throughout 1982 and 1983, I suffered with acute shoulder and hip pains. I had problems using my left arm or walking when the unexplained pains set in. The pains were so severe they prevented my exercising or playing any sports. This interruption of my athletic career marked my sinking into middle age.

In August 1983, during a routine check-up in the hospital, my right foot had to be operated on in order to prevent complications in a toe. Because of impaired circulation, people with diabetes are notorious for developing infections in their feet that sometimes can lead to amputations.

In September and October 1983, I had two laser treatments done on my right eye to combat retinopathy. It would not do for an English professor to become blind.

In December 1983, I experienced my first hemorrhage in that same right eye. The scar tissue from the laser treatment had latched upon the vitreous after the surgery. As the vitreous began to separate naturally from the retina, it pulled the scar tissue away also and resulted in the bleeding. I could not see with the right eye. The treatment for preventing blindness was resulting in what was to be avoided.

In March and May of 1984, two more hemorrhages occurred in

that right eye. It seemed that every time the eye started to clear up a new hemorrhage would come along.

In September 1984, I underwent open-heart surgery again to install three new by-passes. This was not supposed to be. I had done what I had been told: diet, exercise, medical care. I had checked into a hospital a year earlier to update my diabetes care and to undergo a complete physical examination. I had committed myself to a rigorous regimen for a long and full life. I had believed the doctor when he told me that my response to the original diagnosis and subsequent surgery would ensure my well-being.

The promise had been a welcome one—I had vowed that I would never willingly submit to another surgery! I wouldn't face the pain. I could not handle the invasion of a body that I had once been proud. The drugs, the lab work, the scars, and the lonely dark nights had played havoc with my health. It had taken all that I could muster to recover physically and emotionally in 1978.

But there was no choice less than six years later. A "re-do" or "good bye."

In 1987, my left eye required laser treatment. A cardiac first-pass test and check-up documented that the by-passes were holding up, but that the heart muscle was deteriorating due to small vessel disease and resulting circulation problems.

Sure I got depressed. It seemed that every time I survived one ordeal another leaped up and shot me down as I tried to return to a routine schedule. It seemed that the more I tried to take care of myself the worse my health would get. I felt that I was spending my life in one of three ways: 1) in the hospital or the doctor's office for treatment; 2) recuperating from one medical disaster or another; or 3) wondering what the next medical emergency would be and when it would come. I seemed to struggle through each episode and then to sink into a mire of despair.

But now I am done with that. I am no longer looking back into a rear view mirror. I am no longer moaning and groaning about how things have gone wrong with my body and my life. I have stopped lamenting what I may never be able to enjoy. I have stopped gorging myself like a starving man on the foodstuffs of life. I am savoring the textures and the tastes of life slowly.

I am back. I am living my life. I am eating, sleeping, and playing with my sons and my friends. We play tennis, softball, racquetball, and cards. We fish, picnic, camp, and bike. We go to ball games and to movies and to whatever seems like it would be fun or worthwhile. I am working, teaching, and writing. My students and I wrestle with the intricacies of using semicolons and the issues involved in day-to-day living. My colleagues and I are striving to make our department the best group of teachers that it can be. I am moving into professional and personal interests that didn't even exist just a few years ago.

I am back.

I have decided to live.

I am feeling good.

The Cost of Diabetes

PEOPLE WITH DIABETES often feel guilty because treating their disease costs a great deal of money. Coupled with the special medical attention required, the extraordinary cost of diabetes can make them feel that they are a burden to their families. They believe that the disease places an extraordinary drain on their families. They are right.

Consider a typical day for me. My day begins with blood glucose testing. This essential test requires one full test strip (approximately $33 per bottle of 50 which lasts less than two weeks), an Autolet with lancet and platform ($19.95 with 10 lancets and 20 platforms), and a glucose monitor (approximately $150-$265 as a one-time expense plus the $2.90 cost of replacing four AAA alkaline batteries periodically). If the sugar level is high, I must check the urine for ketones ($7.99 per bottle of 100). Next comes the insulin injection. I mix two insulins (approximately $14 per bottle) and use a disposable syringe ($.20 each). Sometimes I use rubbing alcohol and cotton or alcohol rubs ($1.95 per 100). After the injection, I take a variety of minerals and vitamins: chromium for even insulin absorption ($7.88 for 75 tablets), magnesium for my eye vessels ($5.40 per 100), zinc ($3.32 per 50), vitamin C ($4.65 per 100), vitamin A ($2.80 per 100), vitamin B ($5.30 per 60), vitamin E ($9.97 per 100), and a multivitamin for wide range coverage ($4.74 per 100).

After I do what I call "my business," I eat the meal that Judy has prepared. Indeed, the carefully prepared meal is also more expensive than a regular meal. It is amazing how much it costs to eat a healthy diet. Whole grain bread is more expensive than white bread. Fresh vegetables can cost twice as much as the frozen variety, and salads out-of-season truly can become a luxury item. Fresh fruit and water-packed fruit are not as economical as cakes, pies, and such. Meat—normally out of sight for even the nondiscriminating—becomes prohibitive for those seeking lean cuts. Artificial sweeteners run up the food bill even further. If I go out to eat, I am amazed how it seems that the inexpensive foods are the ones on the menu which are dominated by empty calories, high carbohydrates, and fat. The healthy foodstuffs have gourmet prices.

The nasty thing about the expenses of glucose self-monitoring, insulin injections, and eating is that they occur four times a day, 365 days a year. The day-to-day expenses mount up very quickly.

Then a person with diabetes gets into high finance when tabulating the other expenses associated with treating the disease.

First, the quarterly visits to the primary care physician include the office visit and the laboratory work. For me, the office visit costs about $50; the blood glucose test and the HA1C run another $30 to $40.

Then, the ophthalmologist needs to be visited every six months for regular check-ups of the eyes and every three months when some retinopathy activity is detected. Such visits run $45 apiece. If the retinopathy advances to a stage which threatens the vision, laser treatments are necessary. They cost $1,000 per treatment the last time.

Finally, other ordinary expenses include tests which evaluate the functions of the kidneys, the nerves, and the heart. Fortunately, such tests are not done every day. Evaluating kidney function, nerve induction, protein in the urine, and the cardiovascular system can run into thousands of dollars.

Clearly, treating diabetes costs big bucks and can cut huge holes into the financial empires of even the affluent jet setters. For those not of the rich and famous, the burden can be enormous and the resulting guilt can be oppressive.

What is one to do?

I consider the alternative. Like the mechanic in the commercial for oil filters on television says, "You can pay me now, or pay me later." The central idea seems the same. I can pay the admittedly expensive price of daily and quarterly maintenance of the diabetes, or I will pay the unbelievably exorbitant cost later for not keeping up the maintenance. That later cost can be more than thousands of dollars and more than money.

I don't admit that I am impressed by the various threats that I have been subjected to for so many years. I deal with promises of blindness, amputation, heart disease, neuropathy, kidney failure, impotence, death, and other inconveniences by casually reminding myself and others that there are no guarantees and that I could be hit by a garbage truck while crossing the street to check my mail.

But talk to me about the cost of being in the hospital and you have my attention. In 1978, I spent over $20,000 for an eleven-day stay in the hospital. In 1983, five days in the hospital cost almost $5,000. In 1984, a seven-day adventure ran up to well over $25,000. Those bills did not include the tab for the doctors, surgeons, and various other medical people who read x-rays, do lab reports, and perform mysterious functions. In 1978, these other bills came to over $10,000; in 1983, $2,000; in 1984, $15,000. (And they don't go down: the 1978 and the 1984 hospital stay was for exactly the same procedure. The cost had gone up about $10,000 in six years.) Those bills hit after you have been home long enough so that you can survive the shock. Notably, the medical community doesn't offer budget or group rates and are unwilling to take time payments extended over two or three decades.

Talk about a financial and emotional burden over medical care! Even those with health insurance are not spared; rarely does the insurance cover 100% of the costs. Plus, there is the strain and stress of assuring the bill collectors that the insurance company will pay that bill and of hassling with the insurance company over deductibles and what should be covered.

Not only are the primary expenses astronomical, but the secondary costs make a hospital visit even more disastrous. When I am in the hospital or recovering from a hospital stay, I'm not working. Frequently when one does not go to work, one is not paid. When one is not paid, it is difficult to meet the usual expenses, let alone extraordinary medical ones.

Also, other expenses are incurred, such as the cost to the family emotionally and financially. The worry for the spouse and children would tax the strongest people. The disruption of the routine can upset a family for months. The need to visit the patient in the hospital can result in motel expenses, restaurant charges, travel costs, and baby-sitting fees. Frequently, for me, facing the discomforting medical procedures has been easier than seeing Judy, Eric, and Bryan suffer from my being in the hospital.

Indeed, the cost of treating diabetes is very high. The cost includes a financial burden and can include an emotional bill to be paid in the form of substantial guilt felt by the person with diabetes. But the cost of not treating the diabetes can be very much higher. Treating acute problems always costs more than carrying on a maintenance and management program. The emotional impact of major medical disasters can be more devastating than guilt over putting a strain on the family budget. What about the guilt from abandoning those who have depended upon you for emotional and financial support?

After all these years, I try to see the expenses of diabetes management and maintenance as an investment. But I still wince when I have to choke up the money to make that "investment." I still feel guilty about the drain I feel I make upon my family's finances. I shouldn't. I should think of it as a long-term investment that pays dividends to everyone in the family. But I do feel guilty and I do worry.

To combat these feelings, I try to use "consumer" strategies to keep the costs of diabetes down and thereby reduce the sense of it being a burden.

The most obvious strategy is to shop around. For example, in our town, I have found that the price of glucose test strips differs as much as eight dollars, depending on where I shop. The drugstore chain charged the most. K-Mart was two dollars cheaper, but—to my surprise—a grocery store with a pharmacy sold the very same product for 22% less. I also have shopped around by developing a working relationship with a pharmacy in a larger city about 50 miles away. Their prices for all of my diabetes supplies are lower than any I have found in my hometown, and they have agreed—because of the volume of my business—to absorb the cost of mailing whatever I need. Of course, the "mail-order" approach requires planning ahead (I can't run out of insulin and expect my order to arrive the very next day), and I must make a long-distance phone call to place my orders. (The cost of the call is tax-deductible as a medical expense, however.)

A number of national prescription services are available. Advertised in such magazines as *Diabetes Self-Management*, *Living Well With Diabetes*, and the *Sugarfree Center Health-O-Gram*, home shopping services allow you to order diabetes supplies using an 800-number or by mail. A wide array of products are available at very low prices. Many of these services offer privacy options, rush order capabilities, and guarantees of "lowest national prices." They also accept payment by credit card or check. Some even will file your claims with your insurance company.

Magazines published for those with diabetes also can be useful. As well as advertising mail-order houses and particular products and including articles about ways to live better with the disease, they sometimes contain articles about how to save money. A few of the magazines are free; others require a subscription. But, even then, you need not pay the price: when you're at the doctor's office for an appointment, check out what the magazine rack has to offer. If the diabetes-specific magazines aren't there, ask the office people to subscribe. (They can write it off as a business expense.)

Also, be sure to share information about prices and services. You are not the only person with diabetes or who is concerned about its costs. Many with more experience with the battle have advice about finances they will share. I would never have thought to go to a grocery store for test strips if a friend whose son has diabetes hadn't mentioned how much cheaper its supplies were. One way to cut costs is to buy in bulk quantities. Frequently, the price per item, such as glucose test strips or syringes, goes down the more you purchase. If, for example, you are a member of a diabetes support group or know a number of people with diabetes, consider placing a group order of supplies that you all need. On another occasion, I knew that my original glucose monitor was on its last legs. I just let it be known—friends, support group acquaintances, and health-care providers—that I was in the market for a new monitor and that I was looking for "a deal." I solicited advice about the type of monitor I should consider. Fairly soon, I had ample advice about the desired model, information on the company's rebate or trade-in policies, and data on where I could get it for the best price.

On occasion, I save money by making supplies go a little longer than usual. For example, when using glucose test strips for visual monitoring, I cut the strips in half. I can hold half a strip up to the chart just as well as a full one to get the results and thus manage to get twice as many tests from a bottle of strips. (It doesn't work with the monitoring machines.) Another technique I employ is to use disposable syringes more than once. Taking four shots a day, I could be spending 80 cents just for syringes. That turns into $292 a year. I can cut that cost by 75% if I use the same syringe for all four injections. (My fears about increased infection were relieved by an article published in *The Diabetes Educator* which showed that multiple-use did not increase the occurrence of infection.) Whenever I dream up another way to use supplies more than once, I am sure to ask "someone-in-the-know" about it before implementing the strategy.

Ask your health-care providers to help you. If, for example, you are taking medications besides insulin, inquire about generic drugs. If available, they usually are less expensive. Also, ask about doctors' samples. These samples may be for anything from test strips and syringes to drugs and diabetes accessories. On a couple of occasions, physicians—actually their office staff—have provided "reduced price" coupons, rebate certificates, and other information about reducing costs after I have made a polite inquiry about ways to save money. (Doctors' offices and diabetes care units are constantly under assault from sales people from a million companies who leave samples, brochures, and loads of other stuff trying to persuade the physician to recommend the products to their patients.)

Sometimes doctors can help reduce costs if we remind them that diabetes health-care is a financial burden. For example, during one of those periods when I was seeing a physician more often than my regular three-month check-up, I declined to submit to the customary blood work-up. Frequently, lab work is standard operating procedure for patients coming through the office. Since I had had a work-up fairly recently, I could see no reason for the lab work or for the expense. The nurse frowned at my resistance, checked with the doctor, and didn't draw the blood. (Of course, I need to be clear about my motives and to weigh the cost-benefit ratio of declining the test. Is the $10 or $20 test I'm avoiding necessary, going to cost me more later, or something I just don't like doing?)

Just like dealing with the disease itself, dealing with the cost of diabetes ought not to be a passive submission to the burden. I have found that working at keeping the cost down as much as possible has been helpful. First, I have saved a few bucks. Also, I am doing something besides rationalizing about the "investment" of good medical care. I don't feel as guilty.

Cards, Cortisone, and Control

SOMETIMES I AM A JERK.

For example, on the occasion of my thirty-ninth birthday, I slipped into some sort of macho mode.

Wayne and I headed for the tennis courts at 6:30 P.M. for a game of singles. By 8:45, he had thrashed me soundly 6-4, 6-3, and 6-2. I had given him a good game, but his usually unreliable forehand had been devastating. We had had a great time: the July evening had been cool and beautiful; we had had the courts to ourselves; we had reveled in the surprising quality of my game and therefore in the titanic struggle. As a result, I was enjoying a real rush as I drove home. Wayne and I have always been close friends, but this experience had taken on "spiritual" dimensions.

I wasn't home more than ten minutes when Bruce called.

"What about some racquetball tonight? Doubles?"

"Sure, when?"

"9:15."

I knew that I'd just put in more than two hours of hard tennis, and it did occur to me that perhaps I shouldn't push my aging body. But, what the hell, I felt great and unconsciously set out to prove that I was still the man I was 20 years ago.

Bruce, JD, Vince, and I played until 11:00 P.M. The three game scores were 21-18, 21-17, and 22-20. My serve had been hot, and the backhand did not let me down as often as usual. We all were exhausted even though I was the only one who had played anything else that day.

The next morning I went to work no worse for the wear. In fact, when I got home from work, I got the boys outside to help me wash the car. It looked so good when we finished that I just had to wax the beauty. The boys weren't interested in sharing that experience. Two hours later the job was completed. It looked great! Boy, I was fired up. In fact, why not do some work on the VW bug that had been retired in my front yard? I decided to jump start it to see how it was doing. Unfortunately, the bug was crowded up next to a tree and needed to be moved. Macho Man decided to push it himself.

That night around 10:00, the left knee began to ache. After three days of limping around, I began to experience some pain in my right hip. In another day I was unable to move, let alone walk.

Soon I was taking an anti-inflammatory drug. The pain increased. I became less and less able to move. I ended up in bed for almost five days and wouldn't have been able to escape if the whole house had caught on fire. Next came the muscle-relaxing drugs.

Finally, the pain began to ease. I was soon out of bed and back to work. But the medical advice warned me: no exercise for at least three weeks and take the anti-inflammatory without fail throughout the waiting period.

Three weeks to the day I was back on the tennis court—for about 15 minutes. The pain began in the right hip. By midnight I couldn't walk. I started pumping down the drugs. In two days I was in an orthopedic specialist's office undergoing extensive x-rays and examinations.

"Hot tendonitis and/or hot bursitis," announced the doctor. "You didn't give it enough time to heal. Try acting 39 rather than like a nine-year-old."

He recommended an injection into the hip muscle and tissue. It would be cortisone—an industrial-strength anti-inflammatory. No other treatment seemed necessary because all of the x-rays indicated a strong, undamaged skeletal system. He assured me that there was no connection between the diabetes and the current problem.

Unfortunately, the treatment of choice would affect the diabetes. It seems that as a steroid, cortisone converts amino acids and proteins into glucose. My blood sugars were going to go sky high for seven to ten days. A delicate elevation of insulin dosages would have to be made. I agreed readily to the treatment of choice and nodded dutifully about establishing a new insulin scale. I wanted that pain gone, and I wanted out of that office.

But fulfilling the agreement was going to be easier said than done. I had big plans for the weekend. Bruce, JD, Vince, Gary, and I had gotten a cabin in a national forest with plans to fish for bass and to play cards. In fact, in our eagerness for the adventure, we had set up fishing and poker tournaments for the three days—prize money and all. They had delayed their departure for the wilderness in hope that the doctor would be able to perform a miracle that would permit them to prop me up at the card table and in the boat.

We left early Saturday morning. By the time we arrived, the rain was driving even the waterfowl for cover.

"Deal, Sucker!" JD ordered.

We played cards for almost three days straight. The rain permitted only short, occasional forays out into the nearby lakes, and apparently the bass were either on vacation or hiding from the inclement weather. The fishing tournament was cancelled. Poker was the only available action.

The cards were incredible; the competition was vicious. We were having so much fun that we rarely got up from the table. We ate while playing; people stayed in hands while going to the bathroom. I had my glucose monitor, test strips, insulins, and medications next to me at the table. Everyone's beard grew as showers and shaving were out of the question. "Come on, you're costing us money!" would greet anyone's efforts to leave the table, regardless of the reason.

The only exercise we had was lifting the cards. Although we all had the best of intentions, our diet was not the healthiest. We found ourselves drinking a lot of beer, eating tasty tidbits out of cellophane bags, and inhaling turkey sandwiches. We never slept more than five hours a night. The five of us just sat there for three days laughing, scratching, and playing cards.

Each time I reached for the monitor and the strips I cringed with anxiety. Despite my efforts and because of the extraordinary conditions, I had been violating every guideline for the careful management of diabetes. I was certain that this unusual behavior would couple with the promised side effects of the cortisone injection to produce blood sugars so high that the readout would say "HHH" (above 500) every time. Given such variables, I wouldn't have been surprised if I had slipped into coma. I had the sticks all ready to check for ketones.

Wrong again!

Every blood sugar was below 200 except one. In fact, the sugars were usually so well below 200 that the one high sugar (over 400) was certainly a rebound from an insulin reaction. (It must have been a reaction—the way that I was playing cards I had to have been low, very low.)

I couldn't believe those numbers! But each time they appeared, all five of us cheered. Then someone dealt another hand.

Upon my return home, however, I began to wonder why the numbers had remained relatively low despite the cortisone and the zoo-like conditions in the cabin. The only explanation which seemed plausible was that we were having one hell of a good time. Although we were playing poker and they were cleaning me out of my hard-earned money, I was relaxed. The only pressure was to remain awake, to read my cards, and to be wary of my friends' elaborate acting strategies. No telephone calls from work, no cranky cars, no plumbing problems, and no door-to-door salesperson intruded into our play. We were "laid-back" and "mellow." We had redefined "kicked back." We "cooled our heels."

It had been a calm weekend. We had depressurized our lives for three days, and I had enjoyed blood sugars surprisingly low considering the circumstances. In my mind, I had documented again the healthy power of relaxation in dealing with diabetes.

What will it take to convince me of the value of relaxation? Just how long will it take me to implement the changes in my life necessary to enjoy the benefits of relaxation?

Sometimes I am a jerk.

The Fourth of July

THE SUNNY, BLUE-SKIED morning didn't hint at the ordeal that was to unfold during the Independence Day celebration.

I had gone to bed the night before with self-satisfaction. I really thought I was getting hold of the precarious business of managing my diabetes. Before dinner, I had tested my sugar (180—a little high), checked my sliding scale of insulin dosage, and gave myself my shot in a location (stomach) different than lunch (left thigh) and breakfast (right thigh). I had resisted stuffing myself with beans, rice, and assorted vegetables for dinner. Two hours after dinner, I had climbed onto my stationary bike and pedaled for thirty minutes. The 120 tan-and-blue test strip at bedtime had been no surprise.

But the morning's black-on-black strip was. After eight full hours of sleep, I had awakened exhausted. Vague memories of nightmares haunted me. The first test strip of the day had quickly darkened and darkened and darkened well beyond 400.

"What the hell is going on?"

The family's Independence Day holiday spirits began to gain momentum as Judy, Eric, and Bryan bustled around the house preparing for a traditional picnic that afternoon. Baked beans, cold cuts, and drinks were in the cooler; swimming suits, volleyball, horseshoes, and assorted materials piled up near the front door anticipating a day full of friends and fun.

The high sugar haunted me. Why had it been so high? The budding confidence of the previous evening was slipping—no, fleeing—away. "Surely the adjustment of the insulin will take care of it" was more a question than a statement.

At about 11:00 A.M., the second test strip of this Fourth of July scowled darkly at me. My face blackened with the strip. The acid poured into my churning stomach. I fought for self-control and lost.

"Damn! Damn! Damn!"

My fist pounded down on the kitchen table. The remaining holiday goodies jumped with the aftershocks.

While the kids grew more and more excited as the time to leave for the festivities approached, I became more and more listless. I went to bed, pulled the sheet up over my head, and hid. The prospects of celebration held no appeal. I had no stomach for watching people swig down ice-cold beer after ice-cold beer or cram gobs and gobs of rich chocolate desserts into their mouths. No will existed to make small talk. The energy for swimming, volleyball, or even horseshoes couldn't be found. I didn't want to figure out how much exercise would be wise for the amount of insulin taken at lunch and how much to eat. To shoot up—let alone test—in the seeming public arena would be too much that day.

I buried myself in bed as they left for the picnic.

I was aware of my failed gumption, but I just really didn't care. I feel asleep.

Two hours later I awakened. The pillow and bed were soaked. I couldn't figure out what was wrong. I was too disoriented to . . . too disoriented!?!

"Disoriented! Damn, an insulin reaction!" I groaned.

I staggered to the kitchen cursing.

"Why can't you decide whether you're going to be too high or too low? Hell, at least be consistent. Get with some program!"

It was bad. I ate and drank everything that wasn't nailed down: a can of peaches, two slices of bread, two cans of beer, two more slices of bread (but with cheese between them this time), and tons of other untasted calories that I cannot even recall eating. About half way through the gorging—about fifteen minutes—I was able to consider the idiocy of my behavior. I knew how much food was needed to stop the reaction, that I should wait for the symptoms to subside, and that I probably was using the reaction as an excuse for crazy behavior. I didn't care. I continued to stuff—with a savage, relentless grimness.

Exhausted, I collapsed back into bed.

Fireworks awakened me into darkness. I was alone with my thoughts.

"You jerk. Are you satisfied now? What have you accomplished? How can you go into a tail spin in the morning over a high sugar and then go berserk in the kitchen in a few short hours? You're a mental case! What an idiot!"

With the verbal self-abuse apparently exhausted, the despair set in.

"Are the accusations true? Am I also mentally ill? Surely a 'normal' person wouldn't do such things. Why am I so weak? Why can't I just do what I am supposed to do? Why do I lack discipline? Am I committing unconscious suicide? I must be mentally ill."

The cycle of despair kept repeating itself. There was no emotional or physical energy to resist it. The despair led to depression, the depression to fear, the fear to paralysis.

When Judy and the boys returned from the picnic and party, I was sitting in the dark. Even with them there, I was alone. I was wallowing in a mixture of self-pity, fear, despair, anger, self-loathing, and bewilderment.

I did the 10:00 P.M. test strip: no surprise—300. I took my insulin and returned to the chair and the darkness. I refused to eat a snack. An hour later I stormed out of the house and pounded out a fast-paced, punishing fifty-minute walk. I took no pleasure in the exercise or in the summer evening. Exhausted upon my return to the house, I did another test strip. The midnight strip was a beautifully light tan-and-blue—40-to-80. I crafted a fine cheese sandwich and relished each and every bite. I flipped on my study lights and began working on a manuscript with gusto.

I wrote and revised well into the wee hours of the morning. At 4:00 A.M., the tan-and-blue had darkened a little to a still very nice 80. In my mind that midnight sandwich began to taste better and better. I returned to my work. At 7:00 A.M., the new day brought something between 80 and 120. I washed the dishes, straightened up the house, put the coffee on, and took my injection. As the members of my family got up, I greeted each with a warm smile and breakfast. With each bite, the boys looked up quizzically at their mother and then me with my beaming face.

This is no happy ending. I know that this is no way to live. On a day designated as a celebration of independence, I had shown to myself how much I am dependent upon the colors that come up on the glucose monitoring test strips. I had shown that I have surrendered what I do and how I feel to what is supposed to be a means for my feeling better and for being in control. On the Fourth of July I had acted like a slave. Master Diabetes had cracked its whip, and I had ignored my own life. I had turned away from my family; I had not gone to a picnic; I had refused to eat; I had overeaten without pleasure; I had punished myself; I had allowed my self-concept and my vision of life to be jerked around. I had been a slave to numbers in particular and to diabetes in general.

I had enslaved myself on the Fourth of July.

It is no way to live on *any* day.

A Day of Thanks

As I sat at the table looking down at my plate, I couldn't help but compare my Thanksgiving meal to those around me.

The huge plate framed a portion of turkey (three ounces, skinless white meat), stuffing (two bread exchanges), mashed potato (one cup of a C vegetable), carrots (one cup of an A vegetable), tossed salad (no dressing), and hot tea.

My family's plates could not be seen as their meals literally overflowed them: huge portions of turkey with golden skin, mountains of potato laden with giblet gravy and butter, sweet cranberry sauce, heavily buttered homemade bread, and buttered carrots. A glass of sparkling wine guarded each feast. The crowning glory was dessert—hot apple crisp, rich with sugar and cinnamon and topped with vanilla ice cream.

Everyone raved with praise as each course of the succulent Thanksgiving meal came from the kitchen; my family begged for seconds. As they gorged themselves in the best of Thanksgiving Day traditions, I could feel resentment begin to rise inside me.

But I checked the bile.

Before me sat my family. They were the ones who were enjoying the wonderful meal, and I couldn't begrudge them their feast. For once, I stifled the urge to hate my diabetes. I declined to focus on my sense of deprivation.

Instead, I took the opportunity to contemplate my blessings.

First, I gave thanks for those sitting at the table with me. My family smiled and joked and relished the meal. They seemed so happy and looked so healthy. I enjoyed their optimistic chatter, their silly word games, and their unchecked delight in the food's pleasures. They warmed me with their laughter. As they passed the food and teased everyone at the table, I savored my memories of their parts in my life. I savored their assumptions of a future and their inclusion of me in such assumptions. I gave thanks for their having given meaning to my life.

Second, I was grateful for my ability to provide my family the food and the home that they were enjoying. Except for one one-month stretch and another four-month period, I have been able to work effectively throughout my adult life. I was thankful for the modest success in my profession and for the opportunities to care for my family that that success had provided. Despite the medical expenses, we had enjoyed a relatively comfortable life style that met most of our material needs. How lucky I had been: a job that provided, a job that I liked, a job that allowed me to spend time with my family. I gave thanks for a fulfilling occupation.

Third, I appreciated the medical advances that had been made in the years that I had had diabetes. Because of the startling progress that had been made in the knowledge about diabetes and in the treatment of the disease, I realized that I had been and would be better able to enjoy my family and my occupation. Sure, I hadn't forgotten my distaste for medical procedures. But I was smart enough to recognize what insulin, home glucose monitoring, and research on nutrition had meant to me. Where would my eyesight be without laser technology? What about the new research data that showed how improved control of glucose levels could retard—if not back off—the encroachment of complications? While the HA1C blood test could be seen as a threat or a checkup for cheaters, it also can provide encouragement for effective control, concrete evidence of improved control, and therefore hopes for a future. Years ago it never occurred to me that stress or humor could affect my blood sugar. Who knew then that a high fiber diet could reduce the need for insulin? As medical science marches forward in its understanding of diabetes—its causes, its effects, its treatment—I am thankful for what it has allowed me to do and for what it may provide me in the future.

Finally, I gave thanks for those who had been helping me fight the medical and emotional battles related to my diabetes. I have been extraordinarily lucky throughout my life as a person with diabetes. While "compliance" wasn't even a word in my vocabulary—let alone a behavior pattern—I have not suffered as much as I might have from the repercussions of such noncompliance. But, as the complications began to set in, people were there to help and support me. Nurses, nutritionists, doctors, patient educators, diabetes specialists, family, and friends joined together to provide medical care and to sustain me throughout each experience. I am thankful for their training, their experience, their dedication, their care, and their love.

Furthermore, they have taught me, guided me, and encouraged me to be more careful in treating my diabetes. They have shown me how and why it is crucial to be "compliant." I am thankful for their map for a future, for the hope that they afford me, and for the opportunity for more Thanksgiving celebrations.

With so much to be thankful for, I felt very silly begrudging the relative sparsity of my Thanksgiving meal as compared to that of those sharing Thanksgiving with me. I have *so* much to be thankful for.

Crippling Dependency

I AM A CRIPPLE. Oh, I have full use of my arms and legs. My muscles and limbs are well-developed and healthy. I play tennis and racquetball with unbridled enthusiasm. I can walk, run, and play with others half my age—and just about keep up with them. I can do manual labor with my hands and my back all day without much hesitation or difficulty. I always have been physically capable throughout my life.

But I am a cripple. I have been a cripple for decades. I have become more and more of a cripple with each passing day.

I have been crippled by medical dependency. It has been a dependency which I have experienced in three stages.

The first stage is the most understandable. Since the day I was diagnosed at the age of nine as having diabetes, I began depending upon others for help in trying to live with diabetes. Certainly, a little boy in the fourth grade would be expected to ask his parents to help him manage a disease that seemed so very overwhelming. I looked to Mom for assistance with the diet—its exchange lists, measuring cups, and gram scales—and occasional relief from mixing the insulins and giving the injections—leg or arm, regular or NPH? Dad became the guardian of the urine testing procedure and results—"Is it blue, green, or orange?"—and the cheerleader for the prescribed exercise—"Will it be football, basketball, or baseball today?"

My parents didn't want me to become so dependent upon them. They didn't want my diabetes to become a leash or a tether that would link me to them. But it did. The genuine shock and fear that came with my nearly going into coma and dying before the diabetes was recognized made them extremely anxious as I was forced into the responsibilities connected with the disease. They watched me like hawks; they stepped forward to pick me up as I stumbled through the learning stages and the difficult times. "Should you eat that?" was heard so often that I found myself asking, "Can I eat this?" before eating anything. It became a habit to await their decision on how much insulin I should take. At first, I rarely found myself out of their sight. Then I felt uncomfortable if I were on my own.

This growing dependency didn't go unnoticed. When my brother and sister—Jimmy and Holly—complained that "Mike gets all the attention. We wish we had diabetes" and called me "Sugar Baby" behind my parents' backs, we were all distressed with what had developed. Mom, Dad, and I began to remind each other whose diabetes it was and to insist that I take primary responsibility for the daily tasks connected with the disease.

Then, just as I had begun to settle into the routine with some confidence, my father suffered a serious heart attack while out of town on business. My mother rushed to his hospital bedside, and—since I had diabetes—I went with her to be taken care of. My brother and sister remained with neighbors. For three weeks in Baltimore, Mother and I—"He has diabetes"—went everywhere and did everything together as she tried to comfort Dad and to pull our lives together. It was simpler and easier for Mom to do the things necessary for treating my diabetes. I didn't want to be any more of a burden than I already was, so I acquiesced and remained passive. I tried to help by pushing my diabetes into the background.

Unfortunately, this behavior of passive dependence became a pattern for me as my father suffered two more massive heart attacks within the next four years. The pressing demands of my father's health and of my family's financial survival overshadowed my need to develop self-sufficiency in treating my diabetes and inhibited any opportunity to do so.

To reduced the complexities and the difficulties in our lives, I tried to simplify the treatment of my diabetes. Insulin was never adjusted; I ate whatever was put on the table or was available; I overate in order to avoid the nuisance of insulin reactions. I never brought up that I had diabetes, that I should have a blood sugar done, that I should be seeing a doctor or a dentist regularly, or that I should or should not do such and such a thing. I depended on my parents—especially Mother.

I didn't know then that I would have been more of a help if I had assumed the responsibilities for my diabetes. Instead, I allowed my mother to do what she could and to try to push the rest out of our minds. But the diabetes wouldn't permit us to ignore it. At age eleven, I developed pneumonia when she forced peanut butter into me while I was having an insulin reaction. At twelve, I bought the wrong insulin and nearly went into coma while she was in the hospital having my youngest brother, Kenny.

The second stage of crippling dependency was more silent and perhaps more debilitating. Throughout puberty and high school— when the crucial needs to fit in and to belong seemed most important—I pretended not to have diabetes. But the disease still crippled me. I allowed the fears connected with my diabetes to inhibit my participation in the fun and games of my teenage years. I hesitated to go out for football: How would my body react to the extensive exertion? Would the coach cut me if he knew I had diabetes? I was reluctant to get really involved in the dating game: Will the girls think I am strange because I don't eat fries and drink beer? What would they think if they knew that I had diabetes? I would not admit to myself—or to anyone else that I had diabetes.

Paradoxically, I pushed myself, trying to prove that I was just as good as those who didn't have diabetes. I worked very hard to make exceptional grades; I became involved with a wide variety of school and service projects which cut across all of the social groups; I tried to be everything to everyone. I didn't have enough time for my diabetes.

But, it is clear to me now that it was during this period that I was more crippled by the disease than when I was a youngster. Although I tried to hide the disease or hide *from* it, the diabetes had exerted its greatest power by keeping me from doing some things with full enthusiasm (or at all) and by forcing me to do other things for which I had no appetite. I allowed it to dictate my life to me. My efforts not to be "diabetic" resulted in my basically surrendering my life to the very disease I hated.

The third stage of crippling dependency seemed to be the accumulation of the first two stages and therefore seemed to have the most powerful grip on me. First, as an adult who fully understood the ramifications of a life of uncontrolled sugars, I became paralyzed by my fears. I had been playing Russian roulette with my life and the loaded chamber was now bound to come up. Each day was like pulling the trigger and waiting for the firing pin to strike the deadly bullet. Who could live his life under such a threat? There seemed to be no answers to the repeated questions of "what matters?" or "what difference does it make?" or "why bother?" Emotional and physical paralysis seemed the only appropriate response by someone who felt that he had no future. Why plan for the future when there seemed to be no tomorrow? Why work? How could one enjoy the delights of the spring ("an ironic contrast to my life") or the fall ("will this be my last?") or my sons ("I wish I could see them graduate from high school")?

Second, as the emotional paralysis tightened its hold upon me, I was forced to seek the aid of a counselor and then of a diabetes care team. After the hours of conversation about my decades with diabetes and after a complete medical evaluation and re-education, I discovered that I had a dependency much like the first one with my parents. I didn't feel safe without the close care of the diabetes care team or the counselor. While I was more in touch with my fears, anger, and other feelings, the trained counselor seemed to "understand it all so much better." I sought her out at every opportunity to talk. It was a rare occasion when diabetes didn't come up in our conversations. Even though I'd had some assurances that the loaded chamber wasn't actually pressed against my temple and knew five times as much about the disease and its treatment as I had before, I found myself relying almost entirely upon the diabetes educators and the primary care nurses. We talked nearly every day on the telephone. "Can I eat this type of food? When should I eat? How much insulin should I take? When should I take it? Do you think I should do such and such?" While I didn't live with them, it seems clear that they had become surrogate parents to whom I have surrendered a major proportion of my life.

Finally, I have allowed diabetes to cripple me by becoming a "professional diabetic." In an effort to develop a sense that I, indeed, have some control over the diabetes' domination of my life, I have gotten involved in writing about diabetes, making public speeches about diabetes, and conducting research on diabetes education. Almost as a perverse way of denying my diabetes, I have kept the disease forever in the forefront of my consciousness. I have made it an object of study rather than allow myself to admit that it is a major part of my life. Ironically I have allowed the diabetes that I have hated so much because of its crippling effect to dictate to me not only how I will live, but also what I will focus my life upon.

The fourth stage will not be one of dependency. I have seen how the diabetes has made me—allowed me to be?—crippled and dependent upon others. With this awareness, I will strive to free myself of the cycle. I will strive to control the diabetes—not for the control of the blood sugar levels, but for the control of my life. I will try to push it into the background to make it an inconvenience rather than a dominant force in my life.

To live fully I must break away from the crippling dependency.

The Management System vs. Spontaneity: The Case of Sex

I miss spontaneity. I miss acting without premeditation. I miss responding with a natural feeling, a wild impulse, or an unrestrained urge. I need to believe in free will.

I am weary of the pervasive sense that each and every part of each day needs to be either measured out or dictated by the decisions I make with each glucose test, each meal, and each insulin dosage.

If the sugar is low, certain activities seem precluded; if high, extra exercise seems demanded. If I eat a little extra because I plan to play tennis or racquetball, I feel obligated to play even if I have lost the urge, if the heat has gotten beastly, or the kids need to be taken to the doctor. If I have bumped up my insulin, I get nervous when I get an unexpected call to go fishing or to do anything that changes the delicate equation.

I am aware of the things I can do to tinker with the diabetes equation: the snacks to be eaten, the exercise to be done, the opportunities to take extra injections. But a large part of the weariness comes from the seemingly unending demands for the tinkering with the system or for there figuring of the equation.

Am I complaining about a small inconvenience? Making a tempest in a teapot? Should I be grateful with the opportunity to figure the equation? Perhaps, but consider the ramifications of calculation in one very important area of my personal life—sex.

Judy and I have been married since 1968. Early in our marriage, we learned that neither of us was very comfortable with sex manuals. They seemed to turn lovemaking into something like a paint-by-number exercise or instructions for assembling a little red wagon. I recall vividly early in our marriage when we both burst out laughing and said something like "This must be step #4!"

We also learned that we weren't comfortable with keeping

count of the frequency of lovemaking. "Gee, we've only made love three times this week" sent one of us into a dark pout for hours. Even making a "date" for the evening didn't seem to work out very well. Sometimes one or the other wasn't in the mood when the enchanted hour struck. Neither of us got very excited about lovemaking because an agreement had been made hours earlier. When a partner's interest has diminished, there seemed little point in persisting in fulfilling the contract.

I have discovered that for us the expressions of intimacy have to be characterized by mutual agreement and spontaneity. We both have to "be in the mood." We try not to presume anything from the other. We strive not to infringe on the other person in pursuit of our own needs. It has to be fun, not a duty. The more spontaneous the lovemaking is, the better it is for both of us. We talk to each other and try to be as honest as possible about how we feel, what mood we are in, and what we would like.

Schedules, timetables, accounting systems, and competition only dampen our enthusiasm. They seem to be barriers between us that diminish the spontaneity, the communications, and the joy.

The calculations associated with managing diabetes can prove troublesome for such a sex life.

Consider the "let-it-happen-when-it-happens" approach. After slipping the boys into bed, I test my blood sugar before my evening injection and snack. On the basis of the test results, I adjust my insulin, eat my popcorn, and return to my paper grading, the computer, or a ball game on the television. An hour later, I slip into bed and discover that there is an opportunity for intimacy. Ah, what a pleasant surprise!

Then, the little wheels start to spin in my little head and the diabetes equation keeps crossing my mind. How much insulin did I take? Did I have fruit with my popcorn? How soon will the Regular insulin kick in? Peak? Did I take too much long-range insulin in light of the activity that seems forthcoming? So much for freewheeling spontaneity!

Assuming that I can ignore the flashing equation and concentrate my full attention upon Judy, consider her. She is not ignorant of my diabetes. She knows that sexual activity tends to burn up quite a bit of sugar in my system. (In fact, I have joked upon occasion about what we might do in order to bring down the 300s and 400s.) While on this particular occasion she may not know the actual numbers or how much I ate for my evening snack, she knows that this activity wasn't anticipated, and she finds herself asking me if I'm okay or if I need something to eat.

However, assume that neither of us is too distracted by the diabetes' intrusion, that we haven't hurried in order not to burn too much sugar, and that we haven't jumped to the conclusion that perspiration is a symptom of an insulin reaction. What about the intimacy after this unplanned lovemaking? Can we remain in bed and savor the closeness? Or do I begin thinking about the equation again and start to get up to eat an additional snack to cover the extra activity? If I do go and get a snack, might not the lovemaking begin to seem like a "quickie"? Certainly Judy should understand; but I resent that she has to and I resent the lost closeness due to my anxiety about diabetes.

Then there's the morning after when the sugar is over 400. If the only variable is the unscheduled sex, isn't it likely that the lovemaking will be designated as the villain? I am compelled to assume that the "exercise" has brought my sugar too low, that I have had an insulin reaction, and that I have rebounded with what is called a Somoygi. Who wants to experience the Somogyi? Why be vulnerable to the resulting high sugars and the total fatigue? The bewilderment itself hardly seems worth it. How does one relate to the diabetes educator and counselor that the high sugar is a result of a Somoygi that came from a low sugar due to extensive lovemaking? I am a shy person. I know it sounds hard to believe, but a person could start giving up on spontaneous lovemaking.

What about the "plan ahead" or "be prepared" approach? The effects are worse than the early days of manuals, schedules, and counting.

The human dimension of setting something up ahead of time can work, but making intimacy workable doesn't seem to match the joys of spontaneity. Cutting the insulin or increasing the snack can turn sex into a "have to" situation, much like scheduled tennis or racquetball. I'm not very "turned on" by anything that I have to do; I suspect that Judy isn't too thrilled with such prospects either when the mood has changed, the bedroom is sweltering, or one of us has fallen asleep. With insulin absent or extra food digesting, comments like "I'm too tired" or "I have a headache" become more than a disappointment—they represent a medical threat.

Knowing that I should cut my insulin or increase my snack

presumes an intimacy-by-invitation approach. An insecure person, I worry that Judy will not be anticipating the evening as much as seeing it as but another appointment to be met. Who knows what I will feel like in a few hours? Do I want to commit myself rationally to an emotional happening? It doesn't seem worth it if I feel that she may be just fulfilling a contract.

We, of course, have tried to deal with my dilemma. As the boys suggest, after 23 years of marriage, we ought to have developed some "life skills."

While more difficult in the earlier years, Judy and I have talked about my medical conditions in general and the case of sex in particular. To avoid the "I-bet-she's-thinking-so-and so," we have established that the diabetes is mine. Especially in the case of sex, we assume that I will take care of how I feel and of how the diabetes ought to be managed. So, if she seems distracted or somewhere else, I know that it doesn't have anything to do with my glucose level.

While sometimes difficult to arrange with two sons roaming around the house, we have tried to make love at times other than after my bedtime injection. That way I don't have to worry about sleeping through an insulin reaction. Also, if something has gone awry, the daytime schedule allows me to know much sooner: the daylight monitoring is every five hours; the nighttime interval is usually eight or more hours. If I get too low, I know sooner and am able to react more quickly.

Someone even recommended, if only a nighttime rendezvous is possible, that we involve food "somehow" in the lovemaking. Even in the early years, Judy was never too crazy about that idea; therefore I cannot speak from personal experience, but it sounds workable.

More effective for us has been the "case history" approach. After a number of experiences—I've always been in favor of extensive research—I have been able to develop a sense of what adaptations to the diabetes equation seem to work best in the case of sex.

But that is still a compromise. A compromise that remains unsettling.

For me, diabetes at the very best inhibits the joy of sex. The necessary management of the disease too frequently precludes most notions of carefree spontaneity. If I disregard the case history of the insulin-food-exercise equation in order to pursue the fun and the intimacy, I worry about potential problems developing from my sugar getting too low. If I do the things necessary to avoid the worrying, I can forget spontaneity.

Without the potential for spontaneity, the quality of the intimacy involved in lovemaking seems diminished to me. To diminish the quality of the intimacy in my life is no small loss. Intimacy is very important to my life. If I enjoy an intimacy of quality, the quality of my life is better overall. I feel better about myself; the stress in my life seems lower; life feels like it has greater meaning to me because I feel connected to someone.

Thus, the loss of spontaneity is more than a mere inconvenience. It diminishes the quality of my life. I still resent the role of diabetes in this loss.

Silencing the False Alarms

Early one spring I attended a meeting of people with diabetes. During the meeting, an elderly woman with Type II (late onset) diabetes departed from the agenda by launching into a long, detailed account of her current woes with neuropathy in her legs and feet. She was an accomplished speaker. Her detailed description of the painful complication left nothing to the imagination: the tingling, the pain, the numbness, the pain. The anguish in her voice and the tears in her eyes dramatically supported her graphic account.

I don't recall what happened in the rest of the meeting.

While driving home, I had trouble getting the woman's neuropathy out of my mind. Oh, I tried. I focused on the facts. She had Type II diabetes while I had Type I (insulin dependent) diabetes. She was much older than I. She was very overweight. I had no way of knowing how effective her efforts had been to control her diabetes. I didn't know whether or not she had an on-going therapeutic alliance with a doctor, let alone an entire health-care team. Did her doctor know his or her business about diabetes? Did she have other medical problems? Did she exercise?

But my mind still had trouble maintaining the rational assertion that her neuropathy, diabetes, and life were not mine. The alarms went off. I went into a full panic. I managed to get to sleep that night by watching two or three movies on the late show.

Unfortunately, that wasn't the end of that experience. A few days later, Al and I were out in the canoe fishing for bass. Before I knew it, my right leg tingled. Then it hurt. Next it was numb. I changed my position in the canoe. The leg still tingled, hurt, and felt numb. My God! Neuropathy! The woman's anguished account flooded into my mind. I suffered the rest of the evening. Thankfully, I awoke the next morning without any of the symptoms. I waited for days for their recurrence, but my anxiety proved ground-less.

How could this be? A thorough medical examination revealed no evidence of any onset of the complication. A friend who also serves as a counselor suggested that my body had succumbed to the power of my mind. My emotional discomfort with the woman's neuropathy essentially had generated the physical pain. While a little skeptical of such a suggestion—"The pain was so real!"—I grew to accept this interpretation as no symptoms returned to scare the devil out of me. The panic calmed.

But I was not finished with this sort of experience. Almost a year later, I attended a public lecture by a diabetes teaching nurse. Midway through her presentation, she brought up neuropathy. She presented it as a complication thought to develop when healthy control was not maintained. It wasn't an anguished rendition of pain and suffering. There were no tears. The clinical description of what happens—she did not know how—was objective. Not having diabetes, she had had no personal experience with neuropathy to share. Nor did she allow anyone in the audience to "thrill" us with his or her first-person experiences. It was straight facts.

Nevertheless, within 24 hours, I was suffering with the symptoms of neuropathy. Again the alarms went off. Again I panicked. Again the symptoms lasted one day. Again no medical evidence could be found to document the actual occurrence of neuropathy. Nothing in my treatment of my diabetes warranted my anxieties about neuropathy. I had been working hard on my control. I had been going to the doctor. My latest HA1C had been right between "good" and "excellent" control. Clearly, the objective medical presentation had triggered the alarms and resulted in my experience with symptoms like those associated with neuropathy.

The mind is powerful. The body can fall prey to the mind's slightest suggestion of disaster—to say nothing of full-blown emotional tales of pain and suffering. As Norman Cousins has long advocated and documented, a person's attitudes and emotions can have a great deal to do with his or her state of health.

I have to be careful. My little mind tends to wander into emotional terrains mined with thoughts of death, complications, and suffering. Before I know it, I am depressed and then physically ill. It doesn't take much to start the avalanche to disasters. It could be something in the newspaper; a chance remark; or seeing someone limp, use a cane, or hobble along on crutches. My mind can think me into an intensive care unit!

I not only have to be careful, but I also have to be positive. If my mind can take me into medical symptoms and depression, why can't it help me be healthy and happy? As well as working hard on sugars and HA1C results for being healthy, I need to work on thinking about being well. How can thoughts of a future stretching ahead of me, of retirement, of grandchildren, and of the turn of the century hurt me?

With my personality and all of my experience taking emotionally generated nose dives, I will need help generating and maintaining a positive attitude for wellness. I need to look at the documented research that shows the positive effects of an upbeat attitude. I also need to work with a counselor to find a means for finding and maintaining a positive attitude. I have to feel that a basis exists for the attitude and that it is genuine for me. All-too-readily I would know if I was deceiving myself.

I also must work on those people around me. They too need to believe genuinely in a future for me. They need to have full expectations and hope for me. If they don't—if they look at me or treat me as if each day were my last—they can sabotage my efforts for physical and emotional health. All I would need would be to have people asking about chest pains, neuropathy, retinopathy, or kidney function. I would be a basket case. I know I would be—I've been there before.

In fact, I need more than just myself, my family, my friends, and my colleagues converted convincingly to the positive attitude for wellness. If the medical members of the health-care team also believed—and acted like they believed—in the benefits of the positive approach, I am certain that I would *be* healthier and *feel* healthier. If they didn't share my growing faith in the positive approach, I probably would be leaving offices set up for all the symptoms of all the complications they could focus upon. Talking about the benefits of healthy control, of being healthy, and of the future—in my opinion—can encourage healthy control, health, and the future.

However, before I start converting the rest of the world and the medical profession, I need to start with myself. Work hard. Focus on the value of the hard work. Enjoy the immediate benefits of the hard work. Anticipate the long-term benefits. Share the successes and the hopes they justify. Work. Focus. Enjoy. Anticipate. Share. Work. Focus. Enjoy. Anticipate. Share.

So long to the false alarms, and the *real* alarms if I have my way.

The "Value" of Having Diabetes

THROUGHOUT THE LONG career of having diabetes—whether it is for one year or for three decades—people frequently experience strong feelings, such as hatred, toward the disease. They have been known to fly into frenzied rages at a moment's notice or to seethe over a period of years. They bristle and chafe at diets or injections or doctors or ominous warnings. They detest orders to not eat that, to lose so much weight, to exercise, or to test their blood sugar. They would trade anything to not have diabetes.

Strong feelings are understandable. Why shouldn't a person with diabetes feel like a victim? Who wouldn't get sick and tired of hearing about disasters and waiting for them? Demands for ever present control could irritate a saint. Wouldn't life seem more like heaven and a lot less like hell without diabetes? There are probably as many strong emotions against diabetes as there are people with diabetes. Frequently it feels good to hate the disease.

But, is it productive to harbor such strong feelings? They may lead to a diabetes-is-the-enemy approach that sustains a fighting spirit against the disease and results in a rage against compliance. However, such strong feelings can result in high blood sugars and dangerous blood pressures. They also can lead to despair and finally surrender. That would not be good. Perhaps responses like hatred and anger are not the only responses available. Might a more positive attitude be possible? Could a person with diabetes consider the disease's benefits so that the harsh feelings don't have to dominate? Might one consider the "value" in having diabetes?

Yes, the value of having diabetes—the idea of approaching living and the disease with a positive frame of mind and thereby preventing the destructive effects of constantly harboring a gloomy or angry vision.

Consider the possibilities.

On the pragmatic side, diabetes provides an opportunity for

careful health care. People who watch their diet and avoid excesses in such things as sugars, fats, and fried foods will enjoy a better health history than those who don't. People who exercise regularly are in better shape and improve their chances of avoiding weight problems, strokes, and heart attacks. Furthermore, they enjoy a better mental attitude and feel better about themselves. People who go to a doctor regularly improve their chances of heading off any potential medical problems with early detection and treatment. Frequent doctor's examinations and lab work improve the odds. Likewise, those who pay careful attention to their own bodies can prevent any minor problems such as infections or rashes from going unchecked. Also the more people that know about their bodies and their own health care the healthier they may be.

People with diabetes are encouraged to watch their diets, exercise regularly, visit their doctor regularly, pay attention to their bodies, and learn about their own health care. Usually, they are helped with these concerns or are encouraged to seek out those who can help them. Further encouragement comes to people with diabetes because they don't have to wait for long-term benefits as do those who don't have diabetes. A careful diet, regular exercise, and close medical attention help people with diabetes feel better every day.

A second value in having diabetes is that it can help establish a person's focus. While being "diabetic" shouldn't become a label that reduces a person to a mere condition, it can provide a sense of place. For many who find our culture alienating and isolating, diabetes can be a comfort. Diabetes can provide an identity for a person. It can be seen as something which separates a person from those who feel themselves to be in a faceless herd.

Having diabetes provides access to other people who have diabetes. These people may be individuals who are sensitive to another's problems or part of a support group which serves the physical and emotional needs of those with the disease or their families. They are people who care about people. They are good people to know. They are people a person might not know unless he or she has diabetes.

Also, the treatment of the disease can provide a sense of order or discipline for living. Effective treatment calls for careful diet,regular exercise, and attentive medical care—a discipline that many would resent strongly, if not resist altogether. Diabetes gives a reason for doing the healthy things. It also prescribes the way to do the healthy things. It is a difficult regimen, and those who participate in it can take pride in their accomplishment. They face the "enemy" and don't surrender. They "pay the price" through a discipline that few are willing to follow. Having diabetes can be a source of pride because it can result in a demanding discipline that those without the disease can only envy.

A third value in having diabetes is that it enhances the flavor of nearly everything in life. Many books, movies, and television programs show how people rarely value something until they don't or can't have it. Stories of individuals shipwrecked or caught in a desert frequently recount how people came to value things such as food or water that they had taken for granted. Some characters become killers in order to taste a cup of water or turn on their loved ones in order to seize some small morsel of food.

People with diabetes needn't wait to be shipwrecked or caught in a desert to relish the things usually enjoyed in life. Few enjoy food as much as people with diabetes. Because the diabetes diet usually restricts the amount of food that should be eaten, people with diabetes savor each bite: the meat's delicious juices, the potato's texture, the vegetables' crunch. A meal for someone with diabetes is more than something to rush through or to get over. Those without the disease rarely appreciate a single meal to its fullest!

Food is not the only event savored more fully by those with diabetes. Even the simplest pleasures become real treasures. How often is the person without diabetes thankful for being able to exercise or to read? A walk, a run, or a skip is usually taken for granted. Bicycling after work, swimming in the local lake, or shooting baskets is just there to do. Reading the sports section in the daily newspaper, watching a soap opera on television, or plowing through a classic novel for a school assignment is considered standard operating procedure—a given with living for most people. But not for those with diabetes—such activities are prizes. If a person chooses to look upon diabetes in positive terms, he or she values even the simplest activities as something he or she can do.

This intensified sensitivity to living goes beyond enjoying food and activities for those with diabetes. Diabetes insists that people recognize their mortality. While bringing to mind a fact that scares nearly everyone and probably is most responsible for the strong negative feelings about diabetes, the disease serves by heightening the value of each day. While it may sound like a Hallmark card or a wall poster, the idea that each day becomes a victory, a treasure, and "what it's all about" is accurate for a person with diabetes who can focus on the positive side.

The strong sense that the days may not stretch out endlessly provides a great impetus for living. One's children seem more than faces to be fed, protected, and worried about. Waiting for tomorrow to play ball or to go fishing doesn't seem prudent. Many things are said that parents usually keep to themselves. The extra long hugs and the expanded times for sharing exist as regular ingredients in a savored life.

Irritants of daily living diminish in importance. While flat tires, missed appointments, and raised rents remain unwanted, they don't ruin a day, let alone a lifetime. Who wants to waste time blowing a gasket over a temporary inconvenience? Why spend time on anger, frustration, and ravaged senses of injustice? Lamenting over the little things doesn't seem a wise use of time or energy.

For people with diabetes, life can belike eating an apple. Rather than focusing on how that apple might be an apple pie or apple pie with vanilla ice cream, they can savor the deep red color, the sweet juice, and the crunchy texture. Rather than lament that they don't have an entire orchard, they can hold their single apple and admire its symmetrical order and its part in a marvelous natural cycle. Rather than regretting what it might have been, they can benefit from the nutrition it provides. Rather than worrying about the possibilities of it harboring a worm, they can bite into it with gusto.

Perhaps perfect apples exist. Certainly some people own orchards, and possibly others have apple pie every night. But what some have or wish they had need not diminish what others can enjoy. Their orchard should not devalue a person's single apple. In fact, their very possession of an entire orchard may reduce the value of their individual apples; they may not hold each as dear as a person who only has one. The possession of only one apple makes that apple much more valuable.

People with diabetes may not "have it all," but they are not without. To succumb totally to anger and other strong feelings regarding their disease might be throwing away what they do have. They can look at what they do have and value it for what it is.

The Future

THOSE INVOLVED IN THE treatment of diabetes believe in the future. This is a belief based on more than wishful thinking or blind faith.

John F. Kennedy said, "If . . . history . . . teaches us anything, it is that man, in his quest for knowledge and progress, is determined and cannot be deterred."

The history of diabetes treatment provides an amazing demonstration of knowledge and progress. For example, insulin treatment is only a little over 60 years old. Look how many insulins are available now (over 35) and how many diverse insulin treatment programs exist.

The list of discoveries, inventions, and innovations is nearly endless. Home glucose monitoring? In the last decade, blood glucose monitoring has become a mainstay in the treatment of diabetes. Now more than eleven models of meters exist as part of the technology for taking control. Four types of strips are on the market for visual readings of blood glucose levels. The HA1C test which provides clues to the long-term success of a treatment program is a relatively new addition to the growing lists of tools for adjusting and adapting a treatment program.

There are tools to ease injections: some to assist in assertion; others to replace insertion. At least eight models of insulin pumps are available.

The advances in the tools for diabetes care are minor compared to the recent history of medical research. New tests and medical procedures appear daily to aid in early diagnosis and successful treatment. The development of laser treatment for eyes threatened by retinopathy, the closer examination of the causes of diabetes, and the effectiveness of medications for handling high blood pressure and its impact on the body represent but a few of the steps toward the future for people with diabetes.

The history of diabetes care reflects over and over the examination of what has been done in the past and how it can be improved in and for the future. The advances in the attitudes toward meal plans document that no complacency exists in diabetes care. Diabetes care has come a long way from not allowing a patient to eat at all and from the strict prohibition of a wide array of foods.

Perhaps the greatest advance for those with diabetes has been the increased efforts for progress. A growing awareness that diabetes does not yet have a cure and that it is far from being fully understood or managed has resulted in more funding, more research, and more urgency to creating the future. A heightened sensitivity to the problems of managing the many dimensions of diabetes has produced a greater focus on patient education, patient self-care, and the team approach. Nothing seems as hopeful as this new history of an attitude of urgency surrounding diabetes research.

Such a history of accelerating and determined progress in diabetes care is providing a future to a person with diabetes.

I am hopeful.

The Agony of Knowing

No, THANK YOU. I prefer not to take advantage of the unique opportunity to discover if my "high risk" relatives might develop Type I diabetes.

Yes, I realize that I am declining the opportunity to assist medical research, to know for sure that my "high risk" relatives will not develop diabetes, and to avail ourselves of experimental prevention procedures.

You see, the "high risk" relatives you allude to are my two young sons. They are the very center of my life.

I can appreciate your need to conduct meaningful research that may help curtail the future ravages of diabetes. But, if we take the 5% gamble to determine whether or not my sons may develop a disease that has cursed my life, I stand to lose them. I cannot afford that 5% chance of losing.

Yes, I know that a 95% chance exists that we will win and that we could enjoy our lives knowing they were free. But that is a gamblers' fallacy: most assume they will win. To gamble realistically, I believe one must expect to lose and be able to afford to lose.

I cannot afford to lose this gamble.

Assume that you conduct your test to detect the presence of islet-cell autoantibodies and find them. Where are Eric, Bryan, and I?

First, the hope that I have been holding out that they weren't to be victims of diabetes would be ripped away. The dark ominous cloud would be permanently in place. Each day would be spent waiting for the hammer to fall on their lives. I couldn't pretend that I didn't know. Our lives would be changed forever. What if only one son has a positive test result? What sort of stress would that put upon two close brothers? I would feel grief, guilt, and pressed to get them "ready." (Hah! No one can be really ready.)

Second, by participating in the test, I would be committing

them to the research project. A more involved battery of tests? Follow-ups every six months? Experimental drug treatments? No, I don't think so.

My boys are children; diabetes insists that children be adults. Even if either son has a positive test result, why introduce him immediately to the rigors of diabetes disease management? He might have ten years before he has to begin the regimen of appointments, blood tests, injections, diet, and so forth. The occasion for fear would be real. They may not ever develop diabetes. Why start a medical regimen before it is necessary? I will not risk one month of their childhood; it is too precious and too easily squandered.

Yes, I am weak and selfish. I should be prepared to be positive, to accept Fate's hand, to make lemonade out of the lemons, and to offer a helping hand to others.

No. I cannot. I could not endure the agony of knowing.

PART IV

The Health-Care Team

Introducing the Team

PROFESSIONALS WORKING in the field of diabetes care have come to emphasize the concept of the team approach to diabetes patient care.

Whether in a hospital or working out of a physician's office, the team usually is thought to include a physician, a primary care nurse, a nutritionist, a diabetes educator, a lab technician, and a counselor. The terms may vary—a "dietician" may be called a "nutritionist," a "diabetes nurse specialist" a "primary care nurse," a "nurse educator" a "diabetes educator," or a "psychologist" a "counselor." The jobs on the team even may overlap—the physician may serve as psychologist as well; the diabetes nurse specialist also can serve as educator; the primary care nurse also may be the lab technician.

The idea behind this approach is that few physicians are strong in all areas essential for the best possible care for someone with diabetes. Ideally, with a team of specialists working with the physician, the patient is offered state-of-the-art care and treatment. Each team member focuses on his or her specialty. Each has the freedom to develop his or her knowledge of and techniques with the latest advances in his or her particular area. Each can focus on the delivery of his or her specialty. The physician can diagnose and prescribe; the nurse can implement the prescription; the educator can teach; the nutritionist can develop the balanced, healthy diet; the psychologist can listen and assist in handling the emotional terrains. As part of a team, each specialist knows of the important integration of the various dimensions in dealing with the disease and knows that he or she can step back when the treatment program moves into another's area.

Also, by working together as a team, they demonstrate to the person with diabetes that the care and the treatment of the disease requires a multi-dimensional approach. Patients see that treating diabetes involves among other things nutrition, education, and psychology, in addition to medicine.

But, it seems that the team approach should involve many more than a handful of medical professionals.

Sometimes the medical professionals forget who the captain of the team is—the patient. It isn't a "should be"—each of us is the captain of the team whether we want to be and whether or not the medical members want it. Diabetes is primarily a self-care disease. Only through self-care can there be hope for effective management of the diabetes. If we don't have the primary responsibility, little opportunity exists for establishing the essential self-care. If we aren't the captain, all the directions, prescriptions, and strategies in the world cannot ensure our participation. How can any other member of the team really know how we feel, what we are doing twenty-four hours a day, and what makes us tick? If all concerned see that we are the captain of the team, effective patient care remains the primary goal. By assuming that we are captain, others on the team will not compete for the position.

Another part of the team that is gaining more and more recognition as an effective contributor to diabetes management is the concept of diabetes support groups and/or diabetes outreach groups. Their functions vary as does their effectiveness, but physicians and other medical professionals are becoming more and more willing to list them on the team roster. People in these groups usually have diabetes or live with those who do. They know "how it is." They cannot be accused of having never been there or of having a career or financial investment in the disease. Support groups can provide information, emotional support, advice, and a variety of resources. They can point people needing help to those who can provide it.

However, no one with diabetes and no one who cares for those with diabetes can ignore the important roles of the "significant others" in the lives of those with diabetes. Whether or not they are listed on the team roster, they are the first team. The people most often around the person with diabetes usually will affect that person the most. Unless disasters have struck, physicians, nurses, and technicians are seen relatively infrequently. How can appointments every three months or even telephone calls several times a week compete with the daily encounters with parents or spouses or siblings or lovers or children or friends or fellow employees or teachers?

These are the people who are in the trenches, on the playing fields, and in the dreams of the team captain. In fact, they frequently have no choice—they are on the team, whether or not they like it. They are living their lives with us. They see what is happening: they can offer advice and support when either is needed; they can seek help when it is needed. When we need someone to talk to, to lean on, to cry with, or to celebrate with, these are the team members who are most available and most involved. Their emotional investment in the quality of the patient care is usually the greatest of all the team members. Sometimes they care more than we do. Clearly, the more knowledgeable these team members are, the more effective will be the diabetes management.

The team approach to dealing with and treating diabetes is the way to go. It makes sense: diabetes is complex and multifaceted. Future research and personal testimony will document its powerfully healthy impact on the effectiveness of diabetes care. All we need to do to ensure such success is to be sure to include all the members of the team and to honor them all equally.

The following section of *The Human Side of Diabetes* provides a sample of some of the experiences and responses that experienced members of the team have had with me or with others who have diabetes.

On the front line is the first team of family and friends. Judy, Eric, Wayne, Alberta, Eunice, and Liz are just a few members of my front line.

Judy and I met in high school and have been married since 1968. Besides working as a wife and mother, she teaches the physically and mentally handicapped in the public schools.

Eric, my eldest son, was born in 1976. One of the "three puppies" (Mike, Eric, and Bryan), he is avidly interested in creative writing and rock music.

Wayne Dickson hired me in 1968 to teach in a summer program at Stetson University. As well as colleagues in the English Department, we have been friends and partners on the tennis court, on the research frontier, on the lecture circuit, and in the publishing arena.

My friend and counselor, Alberta Lee Wehrle is a psychiatric nurse at a Veterans Administration clinic where she works primarily with Vietnam veterans. A voracious reader, she is very proud of her two daughters—Royellen, an accomplished attorney, and Karla, a successful banker.

A talented artist who works out of her home because of severe allergies, Eunice Maris describes herself as a "family person who always wanted more children."

Elizabeth Pippio is the mother of three grown children and the secretary for the Religion Department of Stetson University. She enjoys "the gift of life and values close relationships with Jesus Christ and with her children."

The many, many health-care providers on my team are well-represented by four medical professionals who also have been friends.

When he wrote his contributions, Marvin C. Mengel, M.D. had been treating people with diabetes for over 15 years. He was a partner in a group of three endocrinologists, was medical director of two diabetes care units, served as director of a foundation which funded diabetes research, and was on the faculty of the University of Florida College of Medicine. Marvin was my doctor until we started working together on diabetes patient education.

Beth Dama Kraas, diabetes nurse specialist and a certified diabetes educator, has nearly two decades' experience treating, helping, and advising people with diabetes. Currently she is the program director for the Florida Hospital diabetes care programs in Central Florida. Beth was head nurse of the first diabetes care unit where I received my first real education about my disease.

When interviewed, Sandy Pollock was serving as a diabetes teaching nurse and counselor at Humana Hospital Lucerne's diabetes care unit in Orlando, Florida. Currently she is in private practice as a mental health counselor.

Linda Ammons is a chief clinical nutritionist at the Diabetes and Endocrine Center of Orlando.

The last selections in The Health-Care Team section reflect on the relationships between patients and professional health-care providers.

The Wife: Judy
by Judith C. Raymond

I HAVE BEEN MARRIED to a closet diabetic for more than 20 years. It is only in the past few years that Mike has come out of the closet and that I have been free to acknowledge his diabetes in public.

We had a long courtship—rocky some times, wonderful at others—and I knew from day one that Mike had the "disease." My earliest memories of "it" and "us" date from a beach trip in the spring of our senior year in high school. Just before Mike was due to pick me up, my mother set a six-pack of Tab on the foyer table "for Michael." That was my introduction to the possible limitations a person with diabetes has to endure. If Mother hadn't provided those sugar-free drinks, I doubt I'd have known Mike had any dietary limitations whatsoever. What I knew about diabetes was limited to my high school biology course which glossed over the condition by making it sound like insulin cured the disease on a day-to-day basis.

Mike was so quiet about his diabetes that even his good teacher-adviser and club sponsor did not know it. The man happily let scholarly, industrious, civic-minded Michael quaff *at will* bottles of sugar-laden Cokes during Mike's sixth-period study hall, which he usually spent in the school store.

During the four years that Mike and I went steady, I experienced diabetes in action. While many of the complications I was reading about—kidney failure, stroke, heart attack—go unnoticed until a crisis occurs, I had plenty of experience with insulin reactions and the accompanying mood changes and irritability. They proved to be the biggest hassle for me. Yet, even during courtship, I found those times easy enough to handle. I naively accepted them as the worst part of his illness. Of course, we weren't cohabiting and my exposure to the moodiness and irritability was limited.

It wasn't until we were married that those insulin reactions began to wreak havoc on *my* nervous system. I have memories of television trays being kicked into pretzels, grease stains on the walls where the margarine dish landed during fits of pique, and the up-ending of a double bed and the heaving of it down the narrow hallway of the mobile home we lived in as newlyweds. I never seemed to be able to predict when these violent storms would strike. There didn't seem to be any concrete situation which provoked them. All I knew was that at unpredictable times Mike could fly off the handle and behave like a maniac only to recover some hours (and a nap!) later. When I would remind him that the melee was probably a result of low blood sugar, he would invariably deny it. There were rare apologies for such extreme behavior.

After five years of marriage, he'd about convinced me that the diabetes was under control, but that I was driving him nuts. Occasionally he would insist that these episodes were completely unrelated to anything except his own unique nature. For a while, I accepted the fact that I'd married the *ultimate* male chauvinist pig and a wild one at that.

In 1976, we had our first baby Eric—some eight years into marriage—and in 1978, our second son Bryan was born. Mike's periodic depressions, moodiness, and irritability prevailed. I attributed them partly to "his nature" or "bad nerves" and the rest to diabetes. The insulin reactions became especially hard for me to tolerate because of the children. It's very hard to watch an adult rage like a two-year-old *in front of* two-year-olds, and then, as a comforting mother, try to make sense of the bizarre adult behavior to little beings who barely spoke in sentences. The best I could do when the boys were very young was to say, "He didn't mean it!" But when they were three and four, I began to explain this "illness" that occasionally made Daddy act "crazy" even though he wasn't really crazy. I helped them, I hope, to realize that we can love the man without exactly loving the "scary" behavior; however, I so dreaded the tearful aftermath of Mike's losses of control that for at least five years I made absolutely every effort humanly possible to keep a sane, conflict-free household.

I dutifully and regularly fed Mike the low-carbohydrate, high-protein regimen recommended in those days by the largely incompetent medical people we dealt with; I subordinated most of my "feminist" feelings, which could be construed as "trouble-makers," in an effort to keep peace; I made exceedingly few demands on

Mike for child care help to spare him the aggravations a pair of toddlers could create; I rarely mentioned his seeking better medical help in larger towns in an effort to get a better grip on his diabetes. I was, of course, still pretty much buying the line that he was "okay" and that "there was nothing wrong." Even open-heart surgery in 1978 failed to convince me that Mike's way of handling his disease—denial—was less than perfect.

I did all these things—rightly or wrongly—until 1982, when I finally could not walk on eggshells anymore. We were three years past our first open-heart surgery; I could see him heavily into denial even after that horrendous experience. He was terrified and had a complete lack of faith in any medical people whatsoever. He had abandoned regular contact with medical doctors a year after the surgery. The insulin reactions—with the moodiness and irritability—went on. We had some wonderful times as a family in spite of the diabetes, but we were a family experiencing wild highs and dreadful lows. The boys and I coped as best as we could.

I began a regular exercise program—probably all that kept me going—three months after Bryan was born. In three years, my running grew from a mile three times a week to five miles four times a week. Then I incorporated aerobic dance classes and, finally, an interest in long-distance cycling. The only times I got real peace (and even to a "boogie beat" in dance class) was when I was working out. The running and the biking, however, really seem symbolic to me. These activities took me *away*: they removed me physically from the pressures I felt all too easily and too keenly on the home front. I knew from the start that the running was more like running away. I rarely ran with a buddy—that would have meant too much togetherness. I wanted freedom. I wanted out of the human race. When I was exercising—and this endures today too—I'm on a different plane. I am honestly above all the crap. It's a spiritual experience. It helps me put everything—including insulin reactions and heart disease—into perspective.

However, a person can't run away forever. By 1982, I seemed to have reached a new plateau in my marriage, in my treatment of Mike as a male chauvinist, in my view of his diabetes. Even though we'd been through open-heart surgery and I had more of a reason now than ever to protect him, I decided to live a more normal life for myself. Quite frankly, I decided to live—period! I quit walking on eggshells. I took off my martyr's hair shirt. I decided to take a six-day cycling safari in the spring of that year, leaving the boys alone with Mike and whatever ravages that could do to his system—nervous, metabolic, or circulatory! I didn't care. One morning at breakfast, while reading a newspaper article detailing the coming trip, I expressed a wish to go. Mike encouraged me— that was all it took! I began training earnestly. I didn't cook a single meal and freeze it for him. I didn't list the contents of the pantry. I packed my equipment, and on Easter Sunday after the traditional egg hunt at 6:00 A.M., I pedaled out of town with some new-found cycling friends, and I never looked back. I never gave their survival a second thought for the next six days.

I think that my decision to stop running interference for Mike and to let him experience more of the parenting role (not just the high points)—yes, even at the expense of two tender little psyches—was a wise decision. I think that it led to his consenting to make contact with reputable medical people and ultimately to take more personal responsibility for his diabetes management. I still stock the kitchen, and I do follow a new diet plan diligently when I cook. But I no longer feel guilty if Mike is alone in the house at lunchtime with nothing prepared for him. He is responsible for what he eats—not me. We don't have many "forbidden fruits" on hand. But I have relinquished my strangle hold on the position of chief cook.

When the children act their ages and behave obnoxiously, I share the responsibility for disciplining them equally with Mike. Before my decision to live, I would quickly and quietly usher misbehaving children neatly out of Mike's way. Not any longer! And instead of harming his relationship with his sons, it has strengthened it. I believe he has learned to exert greater control over his temper as well as to recognize symptoms of insulin reactions quicker, thus enabling him to avoid being out of control as frequently as he was in our earlier years of marriage. He seems to be more sensitive to the frightening effects his lack of control has upon his children, and I think he tries very hard to keep from frightening them. Some of his better self-control these past years may be due to tighter control over the diabetes.

We are not completely without episodes of temper, and insulin reactions do plague us. But I don't believe any human relationships are free of displays of temper. I know that Mike has raged less due to insulin reactions than he had since prior to 1982. In spite of a second open-heart surgery, two laser treatments, and some painful medical problems, I feel we haven't experienced as many extremes in mood as we did. I feel more comfortable in our relationship now. I see myself as a cheerleader for good control, regular physical exercise, sensible eating, and positive thinking. I will always be a shoulder to lean on or to cry on because I love Mike even more now than I did when I married him more than 20 years ago.

The Son: Eric
by Eric Raymond

Hɪ! I ᴀᴍ Eʀɪᴄ. I am nine years old.

I have written this so that some kids can see what it is like to be a kid who has a dad who has diabetes. I guess I should know because my Dad has diabetes. He has had diabetes for longer than I have been alive.

When I was a little kid, I didn't know that my Dad had diabetes. And I couldn't really care less. He would just get mad. I just thought that he was just getting mad. I was sort of just like my brother Bryan is now—I couldn't care less.

But, when I was around seven, I began to notice that Dad was not just getting mad. I learned that he had diabetes. When I came home from school, Dad was at his office. He would come home. He would be mad.

"How was your day, Dad?" I would ask him.

"Fine," he would say. "Everything is fine."

"Why was he mad? Was it my fault?" I would ask myself.

I had no idea. Eventually I learned from Mom that Dad had diabetes. She told me that was why he would get mad sometimes. She told me that diabetes was a disease and that it would not go away. Dad would have diabetes his whole life.

Boy, did I take it hard! I used to think that it was all my fault. I used to think that I made him mad which made him have diabetes. Sometimes I would go to my bedroom and cry.

When I was in first grade only nine weeks, my teacher said for me to skip the first grade. Everyone was happy in my house. So, off to second grade I went. I liked the move. I walked into the class-room, and it was full of friendly faces. A friend I knew was in the class. But, I was scared because I could tell that my Dad was worried sick about me. I didn't think it was good for Dad with his diabetes to worry. I tried to make sure that he didn't have to worry.

Some days Dad is happy. Some days Dad is grumpy. When I had a project due the next day in school and I didn't have time to do it, he would really get on my case. He was tense. He would get mad. He yelled a lot. I didn't care about the dumb project. I just did not want Dad to get mad. His blood sugar would go up.

In third grade, I had a good teacher, but a rotten school year. You see, that year Dad went into the hospital and then had to have laser treatments on his eye. He could not understand why I was in a crummy mood and was not happy. He thought it was because of school. It was because I was worried about him.

My brother Bryan did not know that Dad has diabetes. Sometimes he would whine and Dad would get mad. I tried to get Bryan to stop whining so Dad would not get upset. But Bryan was young, and when he did not get what he wanted, he would whine, whine, whine. Dad would get mad, mad, mad. I could not get Bryan to understand. It was a long time before I told him that Dad had diabetes. I do not think that he understood.

Now, I am not saying that Dad's diabetes is all bad. Sometimes he is very happy. We go fishing. We go on vacation to North Carolina. Dad, Bryan, and I sometimes play baseball or go on walks. On the walks, sometimes I would start to make up a story and then Bryan would continue it and then Dad would. The one story would take up the whole walk. We go on "donut runs" to Mr. Donut at night to celebrate something. I make sure that Dad has coffee—no donuts for him. He and I are very interested in computers. Bryan is starting to get interested in the Apple computer too. Bryan and I usually play games on the computer or do our homework, but Dad writes a lot about diabetes. I can't understand why he wants to write about a disease I wish he didn't have.

You never know whether Dad is going to be mad or happy. But sometimes we can guess. Dad has this little machine which tells him his blood sugar. Usually this decides how Dad is going to feel at breakfast, lunch, and dinner. Sometimes it is low—that means he needs something to eat. He is cranky. Sometimes he gets even mad. If the blood sugar is just right, everything is perfect! But, when it is high, stay clear!

I wish Dad did not get mad. I wish he was happy all the time. I wish Dad did not have diabetes. But I couldn't care less. I love Dad.

A Friend: Wayne
by Wayne Dickson

Arriving at work late the other day, I found that the only open spot in the parking lot was marked "Wheelchairs Only." Irritated, I parked in a different lot and then climbed upstairs to the office, grumbling. To tease me into a better mood, my secretary asked whimsically whether I thought companies ought to begin reserving the same number of parking slots for the "normal" as for the disabled. I realized, of course, that she had meant "non-disabled" or "non-handicapped" rather than "normal," but in a way it was a fortunate slip. The offhand question really did make me think.

"Shucks," I said. "If they did that, then no one would ever use those slots. We're all different, and the closer you look, the less likely any of us is to seem completely 'normal.' Most of us aren't likely even to agree as to what 'normal' means."

At the time, I was just kidding, of course, but nonetheless I do think the underlying point is both valid and important. This is why I also honestly think that, if I were to title the present essay, it might justifiably have been titled simply "Being a Friend" rather than "Being a Friend to a Person with Diabetes." A person with diabetes is "non-normal," all right, but so are the rest of us;and to be a friend to him or her requires no different qualities or techniques than to be a friend to anyone else. The principles are the same; only the particulars vary from one of us to another.

That being so, then, the comments that follow will start from the premise that in respect to personal relations all of us—with diabetes or without it—are in the same situation together. In developing this premise I shall explore a few of the broad, general principles that seem to have worked in my own friendships. In the process, I shall also show how I have tried—with varying degrees of success—to apply those principles in my relationship with one particular friend . . . who just happens to have diabetes.

Please understand that in sharing these reflections, I can in no way pretend to be an authority on friendship or to have discovered any universal keys to its nurture or preservation. I can offer only the fruits of my own sometimes difficult experiences, in hopes that they might prove helpful to others in the same situation.

The experiences I have chosen for illustration can be grouped under three main headings, corresponding to the three general principles by which I try to govern my relations with others. These headings are understanding, acceptance, and accommodation. The particular friendship through which I have chosen to explore these principles involves a man of about my age who has been living with diagnosed Type I diabetes since childhood. I cannot say that Mike has been the easiest person in the world with whom to apply these principles, or that I have been the most patient at making the effort. However, I can say that we are both considerably the richer for having wrestled with our problems together.

UNDERSTANDING

Of the three principles—understanding, acceptance, and accommodation—the first is in Mike's case the most difficult for me to come to terms with. For instance, in trying to understand what makes Mike tick, I find I must struggle continually with two difficult questions. The first involves the extent to which particular needs, attitudes, and behaviors on his part are due to the effects of the disease as opposed to those of the usual assortment of physical and psychological pressures that affect all of us. The second involves the extent to which I as a layman should try to understand this disease which so pervasively influences my friend's life and our relationship together.

The reason the first question is so important is that the degree of my acceptance of Mike's behavior and the nature of my accommodation to it might vary considerably, depending on the answer. For example, I remember when I was in my teens having a cigar-chomping, platitude-popping, profanity-spouting coach of the old school. Coach Mac's standard response to any and all complaints of illness, fatigue, or minor injury was a gruff "Run it out, son! Run it out!" Ill with the flu? Run it out. Exhausted from an all-nighter spent completing a term paper? Run it out. Kicked in the groin during scrimmage? Run it out. The rumor was that Coach Mac had once forced a halfback with what seemed a minor sprained ankle to "run it out," and that the supposed sprain had later been diagnosed as a fracture.

The story of the fracture may or may not have been true—it's the kind of thing kids tell—but in any event two facts remain. First, Coach Mac's training technique was a perfect example of the single, unwavering response to any and all problems. Second, in respect to problems like that of the supposedly sprained ankle, that single response could sometimes prove dangerously wrong-headed or inadequate. Remembering this, I try my best in dealing with a friend whose condition is potentially so dangerous—even mortally so—not to be like Coach Mac, but instead to understand and then to deal flexibly with what's really going on. I can't always succeed, regardless of intentions, but I know I must always keep trying, as vigilantly as possible.

For example, suppose, as has happened, that Mike and I are working hard at some physical task: moving filing cabinets, say, or making bookcases in the shop. Suddenly I notice that Mike is visibly fading and sagging. I suggest that we knock off for the day, but Mike insists we continue: "I want to get this done," he says. "I don't want to have to come back tomorrow and worry with it any more."

Coach Mac would know how to respond—push ahead and get the job done as quickly as possible (the equivalent of "running it out"). I'm not so sure, though. If Mike is indeed just tired, perhaps from last night's wee hours marathon poker tournament, then pushing ahead might in fact work fine. However, if Mike's obvious lack of energy is due, not to simple fatigue, but to dangerously low blood sugar, then pushing ahead might push my friend right into a bad reaction. It does make a difference whether the problem is just run-of-the-mill or specifically diabetes-related—but how can I tell which it is?

The urgency of this first question always leads me forcibly to its counterpart—namely, the question of how much I must understand about diabetes itself in order to be a conscientious friend. The main difficulty, of course, is that diabetes is such a complicated disease it is impossible for anyone—especially a layman—to learn everything about it that he or she would want to. I remember, for example, that Mike was given sharply conflicting advice about low blood sugar and insulin reaction by two different physicians at about the same time. Likewise, I know he has been given conflicting advice about diet and insulin dosages by the same physician at different times. Frankly, I find that discouraging. If even the experts can't get their story straight, then it seems inevitable that the rest of us will have trouble, no matter how conscientious we might try to be.

Compounding the anxiety, for me at any rate, is the nagging suspicion that I'll never gain more than a little knowledge and that my "little knowledge" might, as the saying goes, prove dangerous indeed for my friend. For example, I wonder sometimes what kinds of circumstances might bring on that condition called "ketoacidosis" I've heard so much about. What exactly are its symptoms? Might I confuse those symptoms with similar symptoms for a quite different condition? What should I do, or at least encourage Mike to do, if I think I recognize the signs of the condition? What might happen if I misread the signs and give the wrong advice? On the other hand, what might happen if I keep out of it and Mike himself gets too ill too quickly to do anything at all? It's all very intimidating and, in prospect, very frightening.

Suppose, despite my nervousness about the potential danger of my "little knowledge," that I do try to learn as much about diabetes as I can. The next problem is to determine the kind of knowledge I ought to seek. On the one hand, there's the "black box" sort of knowledge. This sort concerns itself only with what goes *into* the body—by way of food, medication, exercise, tension, etc.—and what (by consequence) comes *out* of it—healthy or unhealthy functionality and physical or emotional behavior. With what goes on inside, the organs and processes that turn the "input" into the "output," this sort of knowledge is totally unconcerned. The seekers for "black box" knowledge will never ask *why* the body needs, say, a certain amount of carbohydrate each day; they will ask only how much, when, and with what probable effect.

In contrast, the seekers for the other type of knowledge will attempt to take the cover off the black box, so to speak. Depending on their degree of sophistication, they will want to know about such matters as where the pancreas is and what it does, what enables the body to use sugar stored in the liver and what prevents it, and how the process of metabolism functions at the level of the individual cell.

All of this poses difficulties for me. By temperament, I'm the kind of person who wants to know how and why things work and not just whether they do. However, I'm not completely convinced that that's the sort of knowledge which is likely to do my friend the most good. I know it would be morally wrong for me to satisfy a merely idle intellectual curiosity about, say, the "islets of Langerhans" when I might instead be learning the relative effects of different types of stress or exercise on my friend's blood sugar. On the other hand, I know myself well enough to realize that this latter type of "input/output" information will be easier for me to remember if I can tie it to some understanding of the body's mechanisms rather than treating it merely as a set of arbitrary and unrelated facts.

WHERE TO GET KNOWLEDGE

Having thought all this through, then, I am convinced that to be the kind of friend I want, I need reliable information. (I'm still not sure what *kind* of information I want it to be, but I am sure I want it to be reliable.) The problem is, where can I get such information?

One obvious source is Mike or other acquaintances who have diabetes—going straight to the horse's mouth, so to speak. Sound in theory, but there are two practical difficulties. The first is a matter of sensitivity. Depending on their feelings about themselves and their situations, not all those with diabetes are eager or even willing to talk about it.

For example, I've known some who seemed embarrassed or even ashamed about their condition, as if some social stigma were attached to the disease: "Oh, you have diabetes. Unclean! Go to the back of the bus!" The person who expects *that* kind of reaction isn't likely to be too happy about a request for an interview.

I've also known those who seemed determined to stick their heads in the sand. They've had to admit that they had the disease, all right, because there's no way for a person with Type I diabetes to avoid that! Beyond that, however, they have ignored the disease as much as possible. They have done nothing to learn about the disease, have never even bothered to determine how to vary their injections of insulin. I suppose they would be described as "noncompliant" (a terminology that has always intrigued me, incidentally, because of the semantic implication that those who are "noncompliant" are breaking someone's moral rules). These persons, obviously, are of little help to those trying to learn about the disease. Though they have it, they know nothing about it themselves.

If that doesn't work, then where else might I turn? How about the old standby, "Check with your physician"? Sure, I can see that now:

"Hello, Dr. Snoodle? This is Wayne Dickson. I'm not really ill. I'd just like to take maybe an hour or so of your time to have you explain all the ins and outs of diabetes to me. Would this afternoon be good for you?"

If I were lucky, I would just be cussed out. If I were unlucky, Snoodle would send out the weirdo wagon for me.

Well, if that's unrealistic, then what's left? I've read some books about diabetes, but I've found them rather frustrating. For one thing, they tend to date awfully quickly, as is inevitable in a field where medical knowledge builds on itself and expands daily. For another, they tend for me to err on one side or the other—toward the black box side, where they say nothing about how or why things work, but instead offer only well meant advice about what to do or not to do; or toward the opposite side, where I for one get lost in a sea of abstruse medical terminology.

To balance these frustrations in the books, I try to look to magazine articles or documentaries or features on cable television. Because the lead time from conception to production is much shorter than that required for books, the articles or features are much more timely. And because the audience for which they are prepared is much more general, they tend to strike a more even balance between black box and technical instruction. The problem is the old "little knowledge" anxiety. If an article or program is prepared for a truly wide general audience, it must almost by necessity be superficial. And so I must ask myself again, "Do I really want my friend's well-being to depend on the kind of knowledge that seems appropriate for an audience with an average education no better than eighth grade?"

The answer is, "Of course not." But how do I escape from this trap? I don't know, and that bothers me continually.

ACCEPTANCE

The second of the principles by which I try to govern my friendship with Mike is to be as accepting as possible of the traits and values and behaviors in which he differs from me. To be accepting in this sense is to seek that middle ground between dominance and submission. It is to embrace differences without becoming judgmental; to encourage each partner to retain his individuality and not to force either to become a "clone" of the other—in tastes, in values, or in behaviors. Clearly, this principle builds on the previous one, because the better you understand the needs and motivations of another, the easier it is for you to accept that other in the sense referred to here.

In a way, the easiest of Mike's traits for me to accept have been those that relate exclusively to the disease. I have in mind here such matters as the necessity for testing the blood sugar, administering the insulin, governing the diet, and monitoring the exercise. Ironically, though, these seemed for a long time anyway to be the traits Mike worried most about my tolerating.

We've never talked about this directly, but I consider it significant that I had known him for years before I even realized he had diabetes. It may not have been that he tried to keep it a secret, exactly, though for all I know he may have. He may not really be certain himself. In any event, the main thing was that he tried so hard to lead a "normal" life that I had no reason even to wonder, let alone to ask. I never even saw his paraphernalia (insulin, injection kit, etc.), let alone witnessed his using them. His diet seemed about the same as everyone else's, and he exercised so much harder than most people that I figured he must be in great health.

I also consider it significant that Mike speaks even now of "grossing people out" by testing his blood or injecting himself in their presence. These procedures seem no more objectionable to me than watching a person drink soda pop or pull on his socks; so at first I was merely puzzled, and I saw no underlying meaning at all. However, in retrospect, after hearing them repeated time after time through the years, I'm convinced that the comments must reveal a deep-seated self-consciousness that was present from the very beginning—in respect to me as well as to everyone else.

And finally, it is also significant that Mike has said, speaking in general terms, that he has changed from a "closet diabetic" to a "professional diabetic." In other words, he has ceased hiding his disease and has begun, if not actually exploiting it, at least wearing its badge openly as a speaker, a writer, and most of all an educator. And again, I'm convinced that at least early in our acquaintanceship I was among those from whom Mike was hiding in that closet.

I suppose there are several general lessons to be learned from this. One at least is that we should recognize that the attitudes toward their condition among our friends who have diabetes might vary considerably, but that many will probably be quite sensitive and even insecure about it. Part of our task, then, is to be accepting, not only of the disease, but also of our friends' sensitivity about it. Another part is to help our friends in that situation to be more accepting of their own circumstances. The ones who are likely to have the most trouble here are those who are unfortunately more squeamish than I about physiological functions in general or about needles in particular. I sympathize with the problem, but I know that if we really do act "grossed out," we are going to be making things tougher on our friends.

Returning to my own relationship with Mike, the reason it is easy for me to accept the behaviors and activities associated with the disease is that I know they are beyond my friend's control. I've never held people accountable for even the most objectionable behavior if I know they can't do anything about it. By the same token, then, those of Mike's traits or behaviors which rub me the wrong way and are also most difficult to accept are those which seem to have least to do directly with the disease.

Among those traits I have most trouble accepting, three are closely related. First, Mike is extremely intolerant of the weaknesses and shortcomings of others. Second, he maintains a sort of "garrison" mentality toward those around him, assuming that they are out to get him by any means available, fair or foul. And as an extension of this, he sees the less pleasant or attractive acts of others, not as isolated aberrations, but as parts of a carefully orchestrated Machiavellian plot. Third, because he assumes that he is the only one sharp enough to see the plot, he feels the terrible responsibility to act as head policeman of his world in thwarting it.

It doesn't really help to point out that these are all simply the less fortunate consequences of one really positive trait—namely, a powerful sense of idealism. I know that Mike's intolerance stems primarily from the very high standard she sets for himself and others. I know that the Machiavellianism he ascribes to others derives from his own insistence on acting with full and conscious deliberation rather than thoughtlessly or in response only to immediate need. But it doesn't help, mainly because I myself err in exactly the opposite direction. I am too tolerant if anything of weakness in others. I always tend to assume that the wrong people do is in response to need or hurt rather than to deliberately evil intention. And I am perfectly content to allow others to "get away with something"—so long as it merely benefits them and doesn't really hurt anyone else. In these areas, then, Mike and I are a continual vexation to one another. I see him as a paranoid, and he sees me as a babe in the woods, waiting to be eaten by wolves.

Another of Mike's equally vexing behaviors seems independent of these: namely, his tendency to act as if he were an island unto himself. For example, it used to happen that we would be at a meeting where he didn't like, say, the business at hand or the direction the discussion was taking. In response, he would purse his lips in silence, cross his arms in negative and rejecting body language, and scowl—not at anyone in particular, just at the world in general. If asked about it later, he would insist that he was merely abstaining from participation and that if anyone was bothered by that, then it was "their problem." Obviously, though, so spectacularly negative an abstention could not help casting a pall of discouragement and ill feeling over everyone present. (Mike must have recognized this, because he doesn't "abstain" so much anymore, I'm pleased to say.)

Certain other behavior is accentuated but not really caused by the diabetes. Interestingly enough, though, the more it can be attributed to the diabetes, the easier it is for me to accept. One example is Mike's roller-coaster emotional life. He is the classic "manic/depressive," whirling dizzily from Himalayan high to abysmal low. I'm sure this is due in part to the regular functioning of his personality. However, I know that it is influenced powerfully and reciprocally by the amount of sugar in his blood. When he starts going low, his spirits become depressed; and when his spirits are down, his blood sugar is forced still lower. It's a vicious circle, which accounts for his having dizzying swoops where others have only a gentle roll.

Another example here is what I tell Mike is his hypochondria. In the afternoon, he gets low and has to eat something for a boost. He complains about this as if it were due entirely to his diabetes. In fact, of course, everyone experiences a low sometime in the afternoon, and many people have something to eat for a boost. (I know I do, and my waistline shows it!) After a hard physical workout,

Mike experiences all sorts of aches and pains. He complains about this as if it too were due to his diabetes or his cardiac trouble. In fact, once more, anyone who reaches his age will have aches and pains after a hard workout. I have aches and pains even without the workout. None of this bothers me, though. Mike's diabetes does exacerbate the normal swing toward low blood sugar in the afternoon, and it does make it more dangerous. And his condition does make him more susceptible to aches and pains, and it does very much require that he attend carefully to those feelings for what they might portend.

A final example of a problem accentuated by the diabetes is Mike's secretiveness. Just this week, for instance, he called in to say that he would not be able to come to work because he had had "a bad night." This put our secretary in a very tough spot. For one thing, she herself was worried because she really does care about Mike. And what is one to think when a person with the following history says he has had "a bad night": a man with lifelong diabetes, a man who has had open heart surgery twice within ten years, and a man with such severe back problems as to have been laid up for two weeks within the past year? She naturally imagined the worst, but nothing was volunteered, and she felt it was not her place to pry. Now add to that the identical reaction by the scores of other persons who looked for Mike during the day and learned only that he would not be in—either with no explanation at all or with the cryptic comment that he had had "a bad night."

On the face of it, it seems extremely cruel of Mike to have put the persons who care about him through such needless and prolonged anxiety. (Needless, because it turned out he was perfectly all right and simply needed rest.) Nevertheless, I had no real difficulty that time, because I know the cruelty was not intentional (for one thing, Mike has trouble believing that people care enough about him really to be seriously concerned), and I know too that once more the diabetes was involved. Put together the fact that the reason Mike needed rest was that his blood sugar had gone dangerously low with the fact that it had taken him over thirty years to "come out of the closet" about his disease, and you will see what I mean.

So that's where I am now. The more Mike's idiosyncrasies are related to his diabetes, the easier it is for me to accept them. The next step for me will be both to extend that principle and to temper it. What I mean is that on the one hand I must remind myself of just how pervasive an influence the disease has on the lives of its victims. None of Mike's behavior is uncolored by that influence, even that I ascribed above to the extremes of idealism or the insistence (in denial of John Donne) that one man might be an island. My acceptance should be broadened with that understanding. However, on the other hand, I must temper my acceptance. If I act like a jerk, I want Mike to tell me about it. And by the same token, if he acts like a jerk—even a jerk who happens to have his jerkiness exacerbated by diabetes!—he has the right to expect me to be enough of a friend to tell him about it. That's only fair.

ACCOMMODATION

Having accepted the idiosyncracies of a friend's values, attitudes, and behavior, it is further necessary to accommodate them as much as possible. Once again, this calls for a balance between total dominance and total concession. No relationship is truly healthy if one of the partners is always giving and the other is always taking. The trouble is, there can be no neat formula to determine which partner should yield on which issue.

My experience has been that everyone has certain points which he or she either cannot or will not give up on. Sometimes these points are absolutely central, as in the case of my friend Brenda's total vegetarianism. Sometimes they are seemingly trivial, as in the case of Cindy's insistence on using the blue token when playing—what else?—Trivial Pursuit. In any event, central or trivial, these points need not even be understood. They should if at all possible simply be granted. Order eggplant instead of veal parmigiana, and use the yellow token.

Once the essential points have been granted both ways, the lesser matters of taste or preference can usually be worked out as you go along. "OK, Ralph. We'll go to Hillbilly Heaven and do the western two-step this time, but next time you're coming with me to that new fifties-style rock place that just opened." The real problem doesn't usually occur there; rather, it occurs when one person's essential point clashes with another's. If those points of conflict are relatively isolated, they can usually be avoided with the understanding that the partners will agree respectfully to disagree. If they are frequent or pervasive, then the friendship may at best be limited in its range and depth; it may at worst be doomed to disintegration.

As I recall how I've had to work through this territory with my friend Mike, I think of three representative areas where we've had to reach accommodation: work, recreation, and social life. Each area has presented its own pitfalls, but also its own rewards.

Accommodations at work fall in two realms: scheduling and stress management. For a person with Type I diabetes like Mike, scheduling is obviously very important. Fortunately, I am in a position in our office to control the schedule to which he will be held. The most essential thing in that respect, I think, is that the schedule be regular and consistent, so that he can establish a reliable daily pattern of testing, injection, and eating. In other words, it doesn't matter too much whether he eats lunch at 11:30, 12:00, or 12:30; what matters is that he eats at the same time every day.

Secondary, but also important, is that Mike's daily assignments be arranged as much as possible to account for his body's natural rhythms. This is of course good management in any case, but it is particularly important for one whose rhythms are so much more pronounced and so much less controllable than with most people. For example, I mentioned above the fact that Mike's blood sugar tends to go sufficiently low in the mid-afternoon noticeably to affect his spirits. Obviously, then, if I can help it, I won't ask him to lead an important meeting in mid-afternoon when his physical energy and emotional resilience will be at their weakest.

The other important accommodation I must make at work involves the management of stress, one of Mike's biggest problems. Mike cares so much about things, takes them so much to heart, assumes so much responsibility for them, that he twists himself absolutely in knots. To try to save him from himself, in a sense, I must watch very carefully what I tell him. I don't mean that I try to play God in determining what he has a right or a need to hear and what he doesn't. I haven't the wisdom for *that* job! No, I mean that while I will ask Mike's advice when I need it, I won't make him the daily dumping ground for my own problems or for more general problems he doesn't really need to be contending with. I know he'll be there if I need him, but I will wait until I really *do* need him.

The other part of stress management is to be careful about the jobs I ask him to do and the people I ask him to work with. I'm not a believer that work itself necessarily imposes a sort of "negative balance" of stress. What I mean is that, for me, getting involved in a big project always raises my level of stress; but completing it successfully and well not only removes that particular stress, but also makes me feel so much better about myself in general that I come out with a net gain as far as reduction of tension is concerned. And because I feel the same is true for Mike, I don't mind asking him to work—I just watch what the work is.

And whom else the work involves! Thus, Mike directs a major project in our department and handles it with great aplomb. However, he was involved simply as a member of a committee outside the department and was going crazy. He claims that he didn't believe in what the committee was doing, but that was only partially true. The main problem was that he was so put off personally by the attitudes of some of the committee members that his blood pressure just skyrocketed each time a meeting was called. A part of my accommodation is work around such problems.

A second major area where Mike and I must make accommodations is in recreation. On his part, the main accommodation is not to pressure me to join him in recreations that he finds rewarding and I don't. For example, Mike loves to play poker with a group of our mutual friends, and I know he would be tickled if I would join them. But I have no interest in playing cards, and I would rather give up novocain at the dentist's than to risk losing money at Las Vegas or Atlantic City. Again, for relaxation, Mike loves to go fishing, and I know he would love to have me join him sometimes on the lake. But I am so turned off by the idea of killing animals for pleasure, even if as a by-product they'll be eaten, that I simply couldn't do it. We both regret this, but it's something we both know he must honor in me.

My accommodation comes mainly in the recreation we do both enjoy: tennis. I know that Mike's body will not always cooperate with the plans we have made, so I must be ready always to yield to its vagaries. For example, we cannot usually decide on the spur of the moment to play, because Mike must adjust his insulin and his diet for the exercise that will be involved. We must always be ready for last-minute cancellations, because sometimes for reasons neither of us understands his body decides not to cooperate. And if we do make it to the courts, we must still be ready either to stop completely or to adjust our rhythm of play to accommodate the changes in his blood sugar.

All of this refers to *what* we must do, but I have always felt that the *way* we do it is at least as important. Mike is a sensitive person who cares about others, and he hates to think that he is inconveniencing anyone. If he feels that his body or his diabetes is forcing him to do that, then he blends resentment with regret in an unhealthy emotional stew. At the very best, his emotions will aggravate his original physical problem. At the worst, he will sometimes push ahead when he shouldn't, paying a painful and debilitating price later on. The best accommodation I feel I can make in these circumstances is to make sure that he knows how I really take the situation: namely, that the adjustments we must make are a normal and expected part of the activity, and that the quality of time we share in playing the sport is many times more important to me than the amount of time or the rhythm. I cannot allow him the misconception that he is imposing on me or inconveniencing me in any way.

The last area of accommodation is in socializing. The biggest concern here is eating, and the obvious accommodations are to adjust both the schedule and the type of food and drink to the needs of Mike's body and not the other way around. This is no problem at all for me, because—as my rotundity will attest—I am ready to eat almost anything (except seafood) at almost any time. The biggest problem for me is getting Mike to tell me what his needs and options are at the moment. As I said, he is very sensitive about imposing on others, especially in a sense imposing his disease on them. At the same time, I am sensitive about imposing my tastes on him or about putting him in an awkward position. The result is that we sometimes end up playing "Alphonse and Gaston": "Where do you want to eat?" "No, where do you want to eat?" "I don't know. What kind of food do you want?" "I don't know. What kind do you want?" We drive each other crazy.

The other accommodation involves entertainment, especially when I've invited Mike to a dinner party at my house. First of all, I try to serve some food that will be reasonably good for him and at the same time reasonably appealing to other guests for whom diet might not be immediately crucial. Thus, for example, I might serve whole wheat pasta, with a choice of sauces and with sausage or meatballs on the side. That way, those who are prudent can avoid the cholesterol and triglycerides, while those who are more foolhardy can scarf up the red meat and animal fat. That's really better than serving a separate meal just for Mike, because it doesn't single him out and—again—make him feel awkward.

The actual entertainment is another matter, and I have never yet worked out an accommodation that satisfies me completely. For instance, Mike used to bug me all the time to get my wife and go "boogying" with him and Judy. So when I have a dinner party, I play records and invite people to dance. Will he dance? Heck no. He likes poker, so I sometimes invite guests to play board games. Does he enjoy that? Heck no. And the trouble is, he doesn't hide his displeasure very well. He "abstains" as he used to do at meetings: ostentatiously silent and scowling. The accommodation I want is to please my other guests without disgruntling Mike, to satisfy all without imposing the tastes of one on the rest. It's really tough, though, and I'm still working on this one.

As I've been reviewing the ideas through which we have been working, several thoughts have become clear to me. First, I have ostensibly discussed the understanding, the acceptance, and the accommodation that I have had to make for my friend who has diabetes. However, at each step of the way, I have been equally aware of the understanding he must attain, the tolerance he must show, and the adjustment he must make. In other words, to return to a point I made earlier, being a friend to a person with diabetes (Mike) is no different than being a friend to a person without it (me!). The principles are exactly the same.

Second, to make the effort to be the kind of friend I want to be cannot really be described even as a "labor of love." It is no labor at all. Rather, it is one of the most satisfying and rewarding experiences life has to offer. I have enjoyed the reflections I have been making here because they have reminded me of how much richer my life has been, for the challenge at least as much as for the companionship my friend Mike has provided.

A Nurse: Alberta

W E MET OVER SIX YEARS ago at a birthday party for myself and the secretary of the English Department. Alberta may have mentioned that she was a nurse, but we talked mostly about books. I promised to give her a call so that we might exchange some novels, have lunch, and talk about our mutual readings. I didn't call.

Two years later, we ran into each other at a university reception for new students, parents, or somebody. Again, we launched into an animated discussion about books we had been reading. I couldn't believe how diverse her reading was, how much she had read, and how vocal she was about her opinions. As an English teacher, I was too accustomed to people mumbling about what they read or merely worrying about their grammar. We agreed to meet the next morning to make the exchange promised years ago. The appointment slipped my mind.

Three years ago, while moonlighting, I agreed to try to a clear a sewer line. It was at Alberta's home. When I finished the job, I had to go into the house to get my check. Alberta reminded me of my missed appointments and asked me if I was still reading modern fiction. My chagrin was obvious. Alberta tried to make me feel more comfortable, but I would relax only after she agreed to have lunch with me.

I showed up for that appointment. During that meal, we talked about our similar love of books, of our similar experiences of moving around a great deal, and of my medical adventures. I learned then that Alberta was a nurse. Apparently, it was obvious that I was having all sorts of difficulties—if not emotional problems—with my encounters with medical science.

Weaving our conversation in and out of various novels, educational experiences, and medical histories, Alberta had me babbling about my father's heart attacks, my diabetes, and my open-heart surgery. Although we touched upon very delicate issues for me, I enjoyed myself. For some reason the meal tasted great and the afternoon had slipped away. In short, we were to become friends. But I had no way of knowing how important and valuable that friendship would be.

As the friendship developed, I soon learned that Alberta was a very feisty person. She would challenge me. Whenever I tried to sweep away sensitive topics by saying things like "I don't care about that" or "It doesn't matter anyway," she would not let it go. In retrospect, it was obvious that she was a psychiatric nurse with excellent experience, education, training, and instincts. But, at the time, she just seemed assertive and intolerant of dishonesty. Frequently, we would get into heated exchanges. Usually I would cross my arms and clam up as we started to trod into what I felt to be a field of emotional land mines.

But Alberta listened and listened. And she heard me. Sometimes after I had mentioned some tidbit about arterial disease or diabetes complications, she would have the full information the next time we talked. I remember well the many openings to a conversation that started with something like "You know the last time we talked you mentioned. . . ." Soon I would have—sometimes whether I wanted it or not—the full, updated information about the medical point and the appropriate treatment. I was learning about vitamins and minerals that were being shown to affect various parts of the body ravaged by heart disease and diabetes, about what effects certain of my sports activities were having upon my body, about the many drugs I was taking, and about the effects that stress can have on one's health. Alberta seemed to become an expert on diabetes so that she could pass on information to me. She bought the latest books and read the professional journals.

But Alberta's focus was not just on data. On each occasion, the information was accompanied by the acceptance of my feelings and was presented as an option. Again, in retrospect, it is clear to me that she knew that my primary problems were not the lack of information. She knew that I had to break through emotionally before the new information would be valuable or before I would take advantage of the advances available in diabetes care. In retrospect, she became a counselor as well as a friend.

What must have seemed like an unending sequence of two-steps-forward-one-step-backward, Alberta slyly moved me to recognize that I harbored a lot of submerged feelings about life in general, about myself, and about my diabetes. Soon, the new medical information and the answers to my questions were opportunities to point out and to discuss my feelings. Over what must have been a torturously long period, I began to discover and then to admit grudgingly such feelings as fear, anger, self-loathing, insecurity, and despair. Alberta kept pointing out that I was practicing full-time denial and kept taking my frequently abusive denial of my denial. (She must have been surprised—shocked?—by some of my language, but she never showed it.) She assured me that she knew I was moving into difficult emotional times, that she was not offended by my outbursts, and that she was genuine when she said I should call any time I had a question, needed to talk, or was having a problem.

Before I knew it—it must have seemed like an eternity to Alberta—I could hear words like "medicine," "diabetes," "heart disease," and "death" without going into a severe depression, turning into stone, or burying my head under a pillow. I could admit that I didn't go to a doctor because I was afraid of what I might hear. I could see that I had expected doctors throughout my life to be gods and was really angry that they had turned out to be humans. I even allowed that perhaps I had not totally wasted the opportunities that life had allowed me. She pointed to my sons, my friends, and my career.

But Alberta wasn't satisfied with such progress. She began to search for the best available medical treatment and to convince me that I had a choice about how my life could be. She found a hospital that specialized in diabetes care and prodded me to check in for an extended visit. I declined. Admitting fear and other feelings is one thing, but overcoming them is certainly another matter. My stubborn abuse returned. Alberta remained feisty. Around and around we went. I wanted no part of choices that spelled h-o-s-p-i-t-a-l.

"Just take a look. You don't have to commit yourself."

"No way. I don't want to know. . . . It'll cost a fortune. . . . I'm too busy. . . . Every time I go near a hospital they want to cut on me. . . . No, no, no."

Two months later, I chatted with a diabetes nurse specialist. A month later, I had an appointment with an endocrinologist who specialized in diabetes care. He recommended that I check into a diabetes care unit. I, of course, hesitated.

Alberta started working on me again. (Actually, she was very subtle. Even if it felt like a jack hammer.) Soon she and I visited the unit to "get a feel for the place." I guess I was on the unit for at most five minutes. Back out on the street, she calmly talked to me about my accelerated pulse, my hyperventilation, my cold palms, and my understandable feelings. We went back up for a longer visit. I walked around—was my back really up against the wall?—and talked to the friendly nurses.

"Not so bad," I announced on the way home.

A month later I checked into the hospital. The rest is history. The hospital visit was not an entirely hearts-and-flowers experience. But now I find myself out of the closet with my diabetes. And being out isn't entirely a hearts-and-flowers experience. But Alberta remains there—always willing to listen, to chide, to "call me out" when I am indulging in stupidity or self-pity, to ask "what's up?"

I now believe that Alberta's role has been one of the most significant—if not the most significant—in helping me to turn around my life. She prepared me—she would say that I prepared myself—to take advantage of the advances in diabetes care. Before I could start doing the important things in order to deal with diabetes as a physical disease—seeing a doctor regularly, learning about the disease, monitoring the blood sugars, adjusting the insulin, following the diet, exercising sensibly—I had to deal with the emotional terrains inherent in my relationship with my diabetes. Alberta gave me the courage to ask and to try to answer such questions as "Am I worth saving?" "Am I willing to have hope?" "Am I willing to make a choice?" "Can I give myself permission to be human?" and "Will I allow myself to be vulnerable enough to embark on such a medical and emotional journey?"

I still don't have all the answers—and I may never—and life with diabetes is still no frolic in the park. But I do know that without an Alberta—without some sort of counselor on the team—I had little chance of turning around my attitude toward life with the disease. Furthermore, I don't think that I could sustain the strength and the energy necessary to keep waging the battle against diabetes without someone to help me with the feelings that come with it. A counselor—whether a psychiatric nurse, a psychologist, a social worker, or just a sensitive someone—is, in a word, *vital*. For me, without a person such as Alberta on the health-care team, the other members would be virtually useless. I would never have met them, let alone taken advantage of their respective expertise. I needed to know myself better, and to do that I needed someone to listen to me, to hear me, and to help me.

Alberta did those things for me and continues to do them. She is an honest, authentic, and dedicated counselor who puts the "patient's" welfare above all. She also is a good friend who knows her modern fiction.

A Mother of a Child with Diabetes: Eunice
by Eunice Maris

I PANICKED WHEN TOLD that my son Eric had developed diabetes. He was only nine years old. Isn't diabetes a disease for old people? Hospital scenes of people suffering with kidney failure, blindness, and amputations came to mind then.

Now, after more than a decade, more personal scenes gnaw at me. One such scene developed quite early. Upon diagnosis, Eric was admitted immediately to the hospital, and the three of us were promptly educated about diabetes. We came to understand the condition; we learned to test his urine; we learned how to administer the insulin. We also learned—from the hospital staff and from recordings of a variety of famous athletes and actors—that Eric could lead a *normal* life with diabetes. Eric was discharged from the hospital—to a life that has been anything BUT normal. I'll never forget that crucial initial deception.

Another scene that dominates my recollections of Eric's experiences with diabetes is his camp experience. At the age of ten, Eric trundled off to summer camp with more than one hundred other children who had diabetes. I would recommend the experience and the program for parent and child alike. The child gets to see that other children share similar experiences with a chronic disease. Parent and child learn that the child can survive apart from the family. Parents can enjoy some relief from that diabetes schedule for two weeks. Customary camp activities shared the children's schedules with blood tests, eye examinations, and learning how to give themselves their injections. A great deal of teaching, counseling, and encouraging accompanied the laughter and fun. The staff promoted regular exercise and a diet of moderation. Any diet, in their approach, was okay—except sugared soft drinks—as long as nothing was eaten to excess. I remember well my discomfort with such an approach to a diabetes diet. The discomfort turned to distress with their entire approach when the staff kept telling us and reminding us that children with diabetes could lead NORMAL lives. The year that we had been living with diabetes just hadn't been the normal year of a child's life.

A third scene which remains vivid actually is a chaotic collage of Eric's adolescence. Eric's early years had not been too difficult for us as parents of a child with a disease requiring vigilance: we were still overseers, were accepted as such by my son, and were able to expect cooperation in managing his diabetes. But the teenage years for Eric, as for most adolescents attempting to grow up, brought rebelliousness and indifference. We were never quite sure how to handle Eric's use or abuse of his diabetes as a vehicle for his rebellion. We were never quite sure how to deal with a "situation." It was a time when we should have been able to give him more control over his own life—for him to make some of his own decisions and to become more self-reliant. It wasn't working: he wasn't meeting his responsibilities. Teachers pressed us to demand more from Eric in his schoolwork and to make sure that he didn't miss so many days of school. It was so frustrating! He was well-liked, had many friends, and was outgoing. He was bright, but refused to apply himself in his schoolwork, his music, and sports. It just seemed that he was wasting such talent. Of course, we worked with counselors and with Eric as a teenager who was having some difficulties handling the pressures of growing up.

But, I suspect that more might have been done with Eric as a teenager with diabetes. Furthermore, I fear that Eric's teenage problems were rooted in an unfortunate history with the school system regarding his diabetes. His teachers, in my opinion, fell short in trying to understand the problems of diabetes and were therefore incapable or unwilling to do their part in helping the child with diabetes. In the fourth grade, Eric was made to go into a dark coat closet to have his 10:00 A.M. snack. It was months later before he revealed that he was made to feel guilty. When we insisted that he not be sent out to have his snack, the teacher made it clear that she was very unhappy. She never made any attempts to hear or to understand anything about diabetes. In the eleventh grade, Eric struggled with a fluctuating metabolism, was sick a lot with complications, missed about one-third of school, and was hospitalized nine times. The school was uninterested in "why" he missed school—they just said it had to stop. We were made to feel like accomplices in creating excuses for his "truancy." When Eric did go to school, they pressured him to shape up. Of course, the more they pressured the more he rebelled.

In contrast, the doctors were advising us to "let up, " to ease off on the pressure, to give him more freedom, and to leave the decision-making to him. They warned that there would be serious consequences otherwise. We tried their way. The result? Even more sickness, more hospitalization, and more days of school missed. He did not test his urine; he wouldn't get enough rest; he consumed far too much sugar; he was rarely regulated. What were we to do? We vacillated from one approach to another. Finally, we felt we had to return to a more parental role, even to watching him actually do his urine tests. Oh, we hated this policeman role. But what choice did we have if he was to avoid further serious illness?

We were terrified. We had already seen Eric taken in an ambulance to the hospital in a coma. The only other child with diabetes in our town we knew about had just died from diabetes complications. Also, we had learned that two children Eric had known at summer camp had died. It had pained us to overhear Eric talking with a friend discussing the two deaths and speculating whether the deaths were suicide and whether it was worthwhile to adhere to all the precautions that diabetes demands. He was so fatalistic! He sounded like a tired old man so weary of life.

That collage of experiences is so painful to recall. We never knew how to deal with the chaos. I wish that there had been a support group where we could share information, experiences, and our feelings. We felt so alone. Just more information could have helped us to diminish our anxieties, frustrations, and feelings of guilt in dealing with our child-adolescent-man.

I now know that we were not alone. In fact, the fourth scene that rushes to my mind showed me several years ago that lots of parents had experienced difficult times while their children suffered with diabetes. When Eric was sixteen, a young minister brought us a bag of syringes, some insulin, and some other diabetes paraphernalia. The minister was being thoughtful because he knew Eric could use them, but the occasion for his thoughtfulness was devastating. He told us that a twenty-two year old girl with diabetes no longer needed them: she had committed suicide. She had become a part of the unusually high suicide rate among teenagers with diabetes. Many with diabetes tend to get very depressed because they feel they are living a strict life that has too many rules, too high expectations, and too many people distributing life-or-death advice. Many are unable to handle the pressure of constant anxiety about dying or suffering with the complications of a seemingly relentless disease. Had the parents of that twenty-two-year-old worried her too much about urine tests, diet, and injections? Had they been worrying her less than we were Eric? More? Who could not be afraid that his or her son also might become one of the horrible statistics? What about not worrying your child about the diabetes? What if parents leave the child alone to "develop maturity and to assume the responsibility" and the child declines to assume that role? Isn't the child committing suicide in a slower way?

I guess that it is only in recent years that we have come to realize that we feel betrayed by the doctors. Over the years we have learned that a person with diabetes does NOT lead a *normal* life. This is not to say that Eric didn't enjoy most aspects of life as others do, but I question the wisdom of constantly telling children who have diabetes and their parents that life is or will be *normal*. It sets up false expectations for them and can result in their questioning the other things that the doctors tell them. With the diet, sugar tests, and the rest, how could anyone say that that's a normal life? I have never seen the diabetes regimen in a situation comedy on television depicting the normal American family life. When we realize that it won't be normal, we can't help but wonder what else did they tell us that isn't accurate?

Furthermore, there have been times when we did not feel comfortable with the information—or the lack of information—given by the doctors. We have had occasion for this concern. When Eric was eight years old, he had an accident in which he was severely burned. When we took him to the hospital, the attending physician found sugar in Eric's urine and asked if our families had a history of diabetes. When told that Eric was adopted, the doctor said not to worry about it and that the sugar was probably the pancreas' reaction to the accident. Eric was transferred to another hospital for a series of plastic surgery operations. They were to repair the damage from third degree burns. When we asked the surgeon about possible complications due to the sugar in Eric's urine, he was astonished. None of the reports he had received contained that vital piece of information! In fact, he assumed we were mistaken; surely, if there had been sugar, the information would have been forwarded. Eric spent the entire summer in the hospital, and no one bothered to check his sugar levels. We were not even warned or informed about any symptoms to watch for in the future.

By age nine, Eric had begun to experience chronic bedwetting, extreme fatigue, and an insatiable thirst. A neighbor happened to mention one day that while at work she had seen Eric's medical records and said that they clearly stated the presence of sugar in his urine. She urged us to get Eric to the doctor immediately. This resulted in the fateful diagnosis and my panicked flood of initial scenes regarding diabetes. (Coincidentally, this caring and informing neighbor lost her eyesight. She was a young mother who had diabetes. A year later, she lost one leg and then another. Then she died.) To this day, I believe that the diagnosis was over a year late and that the doctors had allowed Eric to undergo the unsavory experiences of diabetes onset unnecessarily. And I worry that that delay may have contributed to pushing Eric down the very same road that our helpful neighbor had gone down.

So I suffer with my own scenes about diabetes. One of the most frustrating aspects of rearing our son who has diabetes is a question with which we still struggle: To what extent were Eric's problems connected to his diabetes? Was it the diabetes or his personality or simply the normal (I hate that word!) growth pains that seemed to make his life so miserable? We never knew how to respond. Even now, as Eric is out on his own and a father himself, we do not know. The question still exists. So do some of the problems. I still worry and fear that more painful scenes related to diabetes and my son will be ingrained in my memory.

Another Mother of a Child
With Diabetes: Liz
by Elizabeth Pippio

I REMEMBER BEING A TEENAGER and watching my mother grow increasingly ill as days went by and finally hearing that she had diabetes. With that discovery, I remembered stories of my grandmother having diabetes, having a leg amputated, and eventually dying from diabetes. I recall feeling sick all over and wanting to run out of the house when I overheard the news about my mother. I loved my mother very much, so much so that she was the single most important person in my life. I couldn't bear the thought of this dread disease taking my mother from me.

My mother was put on insulin from the very beginning, and I would wince watching her inject herself. I suffered with her throughout her ordeal with the disease. Eventually, my greatest fear was realized: the diabetes did take my mother from me. I was seventeen when she died, and I was thrown into the position as head of the household. I also felt alone.

That background gave me my mental picture of diabetes. There is little doubt that it influenced my frame of mind when Laura's diagnosis was made.

So many years ago but seemingly just yesterday, we had just sold our home, had moved to a rental, and finally moved again into our new home. Things were hectic and emotionally charged with just the moving, but we also were starting adoption procedures for a cousin who had been abused.

During this turmoil, our pediatrician had taken a urine sample as part of a checkup for our four-year-old Laura. The positive urine test caused him to order further tests. Thank God, he had recalled the history of diabetes in the family. I feel we were blessed because we were spared the stress of a newly-diagnosed child having to reach severe illness or coma before the diabetes was detected.

Laura was admitted to Variety Children's Hospital in Miami. A wonderful pediatric endocrinologist—Dr. Rafael Bjar—told us what we had been prepared for. I wish I could aptly convey what the impact of those words had on me at the time. The doctor might as well as have said that my daughter had cancer or leprosy—it was that hard to hear! I don't recall what was said for the next hour and a half as my mind raced in a million different directions. I knew enough about diabetes to be terrified for my little girl, and I knew I knew nothing about how to care for her.

In no time, Laura was to go home. This meant that I had to show the doctor that I could give her an injection. I had been given an orange to practice on. Heck, a piece of cake! I soon felt confident that I would have no problem with that much of Laura's care. The day Laura was to leave the hospital Dr. Bejar called me to the nurses' station to talk with me. Then he handed me a syringe filled with saline solution and told me to inject him. I pretended to be calm, imagined that he was an orange, and injected the good doctor. He turned to smile with approval as I collapsed to the floor in a dead faint. Some nurse I would be for Laura!

Once home, Laura experienced a "honeymoon" period when the need for injections was delayed. I now feel that God was protecting not only Laura, but also was allowing me to get ready emotionally for the inevitable day when Laura would have to go on insulin.

The honeymoon lasted two months. Despite Laura's strict diet, Laura's urine tests showed a need for insulin. Dr. Bejar asked me if I would like to bring Laura to his office for her first shot. That sounded great, but then I asked him, "What about tomorrow and the next day and the next?" That was what he wanted to hear. He was delighted that I had thought things through. He said, "You both are going to be all right."

I shall never forget that first shot. Laura's little face looking up at me with wide-eyed innocence and trust, and my trying so hard to be calm and collected! I did some praying for strength. She never shed a tear, and we hugged each other when it was over. (I had turned away so that she would not see my tears.)

Once Ed and I had recovered from the initial shock of Laura's diagnosis, we started to seek all the available information we could get our hands on in order for us to become educated about diabetes.

We are most thankful for the long discussions with Dr. Bejar who willingly shared his vast experiences with us. The Juvenile Diabetes Foundation responded to our inquiries, and we spent hours reading articles about diabetes and the physical and emotional adjustments we all would have to make.

Several years went by with relative ease. Laura was on one injection a day. Due to her young age, she cooperated by following her diet. She ate what Mommy put in front of her. Even holidays then were not an ordeal: family and friends went out of their way to provide my little girl with sugarless goodies. I have always been touched by those who were sensitive to Laura's needs to be like the other kids.

When Laura entered elementary school, we notified the school office and her teachers of her diabetes. We supplied them with written information about what to do if she exhibited behavior which might indicate an insulin reaction or a pre-coma condition. We stressed the importance of Laura having her scheduled snacks and of not rewarding her with candy or other such treats.

What we hadn't planned on was Laura's not wanting her friends to know that she had diabetes. She—as a seven-year-old—had learned all too soon that some children could be cruel. They would say things like, "Oh, don't touch me! I don't want to catch diabetes!" Laura would come home in tears, asking if what she had was "catchable."

Such experiences revealed to me that being a mother had more roles if one of your children has diabetes. Besides cook, caretaker, listener, disciplinarian, companion, referee, activities director, and chauffeur, I also found myself being a nurse and a psychologist. I had to become acquainted with medical terminology, the mechanics of diabetes, and the complications that come during a simple illness. I would lie in bed at night with my head spinning from all the data flooding my mind: dosage adjustment, urine testing, diet control, and insulin reactions. I also had to learn how to handle effectively the emotional spin-offs from living with the disease. Was Laura's personality shift due to a low blood sugar? Was she lethargic because she is tired or because her sugar is too high?

I wondered if I would ever come to grips with this new and imposing disease. I would feel momentary victory in one area of diabetes management only to experience defeat in another.

I think Laura also wondered. As she grew older and more accustomed to her new life style, I thought it would be good for her to give herself her injections. By age seven, she had learned to test her urine, to calibrate the insulin, and to draw up the insulin in the syringe. But she refused to give herself the shot.

As the idea of her giving herself her injections began to become an "issue," our new physician recommended that Laura go to a diabetes summer camp. It was to be two weeks with counselors, medical staff, and other children with diabetes. We hoped that she would enjoy the fun, the education, and the sharing of a common problem with others. Watching her wave goodbye from the departing bus was probably the hardest thing that my husband and I had ever had to do. Two weeks would seem like a lifetime.

Laura wrote to us from camp. She told of her new friends and of the new things she was learning. At the bottom of that first letter, she had added, "Don't tell anyone, but today I gave myself my first shot." I think Ed and I cried for over fifteen minutes.

As with any child, one year melted into another. For the most part, we had little difficulty in managing all that was needed to be done daily. Laura was growing a little slower than most children her age, but the doctor said that this was common for children with diabetes. All three of our children had developed a remarkable closeness; we were quite a happy young family!

Then one Halloween disrupted it all. All the kids were excited about their costumes and their thoughts of bags of goodies. The whole day—in and out of school—had been one of festivities. Trying to get the children calmed down enough for baths and bed had been a chore. Finally, we heard prayers, tucked their little bodies in, and kissed cheeks good night: apparently peace had returned to our home long last.

Ed and I were awakened from a deep sleep by the most horrible screaming we had ever heard. Laura was in a grand mal seizure. Her little body was convulsing and rigid. Oh, the scream—that horrible scream! We didn't know what was happening. We didn't know what to do. I dialed 911. It seemed like an eternity before the ambulance arrived.

At the hospital, the doctor told us that Laura had had a severe insulin reaction. She was released in a few days, and things returned to relative quiet.

Again, in the middle of the night, the deafening screams awakened us. Before Ed could get her to the kitchen to administer instant glucose, Laura began to turn blue. Ed gave mouth-to-mouth resuscitation until the paramedics arrived.

This scene was repeated several more times within the next several weeks. Our doctor was at a loss to explain the seizures. But it wasn't due to a lack of effort. He conducted hours of reading research, held long distance conversations with other physicians, and attended meetings of diabetes specialists. I took Laura to specialists. An EEG after the latest attack had indicated some brain dysfunction.

Finally, our physician concluded that Laura was suffering due to a Somoygi Effect or rebound phenomenon. A whole new set of words and new thinking! Back to my reading and research. Apparently, while testing her urine at night, Laura seemed to be having a high reading. What we didn't know was that the sugar was high due to an insulin reaction. To compensate for the high sugar, we had been increasing her morning dosage. We thought that she didn't have enough insulin in the morning. In fact, she had had too much insulin and was having insulin reactions which had caused her liver to kick in stored sugars. By bumping up her dosages, we were causing ever more severe reactions. How could we have known?

This was complicated further by some apparent brain damage during the early insulin reactions. The damaged brain had subsequently begun to send out erratic signals during the later insulin reactions. These erratic signals had caused the grand mal seizures. That's how I remember it, but, considering my state of mind throughout this ordeal, I couldn't guarantee the accuracy of the medical knowledge.

Laura went to two shots a day and phenobarbital three times a day. We had some problems adjusting both dosages—she had some trouble staying awake—but the seizures stopped. Nevertheless, it was four years before Laura, Ed, or I could sleep through an entire night. We would get up at midnight and 3:00 A.M. to test her urine and to give her a snack if necessary.

Once again, Laura took it all in stride and never complained. In fact, she managed to be at the top of her class throughout grade school. She participated in gymnastics, dance, cheerleading, and all the activities at school.

For us at home, it was not as simple. We had two other children who desperately needed our attention and time also. How could we keep the anxiety level down and hide our constant concern? Also

Laura needed to know that she wouldn't be allowed to use her disease as a tool for manipulation or punishment of her parents to get what she wanted. But, Marie and Tony needed to be sensitive and understanding without building up resentment and hostility because of what to be unequal sharing of our time and energy.

Furthermore, not all problems at home were external or Laura's. As her mother, I felt responsible for Laura's seizure disorder. Boy, I whipped myself with that guilt for months! As her father, Ed reacted with feelings of hopelessness and frustration. On occasion he would yell at me, "Why did you allow this happen?" "What did you let her eat?" or "Did you forget to give her her bedtime snack?" That not only contributed to my guilt, but also increased the tension around the house. Although I seemed externally calm and in control, I suffered with remorse and guilt.

By the time Laura was in the fifth grade, she still would not discuss diabetes nor did she want people at school to know of her disease. She didn't want to be "different." I was no child psychologist. How could I listen and tell her she was no different and then insist on her following her diabetes schedule?

Because of our fear of insulin reactions and seizures, slumber parties at friends' homes were out. Maybe some day? We tried to compensate by having several at our home. Once we relented . . . and regretted it. Close friends called early that morning hysterically screaming that Laura was having a convulsion. I confess that I was glad someone else had had to live through such an ordeal. At least someone else knew that scream of a child—that pit of hell I had experienced.

But we were lucky. This emotional turmoil seemed to turn around for all of us. We became active in the Juvenile Diabetes Foundation, assisting in fund raising and attending meetings. Laura was chosen JDF national poster child. Before we knew it, we were besieged by newspaper reporters and photographers. Laura's picture and story appeared in the newspapers everywhere.

Laura's secret was out. When she got to school, her classmates were so excited. They had seen her picture in the local papers and had read the story. Poor Laura, she was so embarrassed! Fortunately, her teacher saw what was happening and sent her on errands throughout the school. In her absence, Mrs. Politis put the poster up on the board, displayed some of the articles, and invited a class discussion about diabetes.

Upon her return to class, Laura discovered a whole new attitude toward diabetes and her. No longer was Laura the object of jokes and ignorant remarks in her class. They were anxious to hear what Laura had to share and were proud of someone who could give herself shots and not cry. From that day on, Laura seemed to exhibit a new attitude toward herself and her disease.

The years were swiftly slipping by us. One day we had toddlers, and the next we faced three teenagers getting ready for high school. The town we had enjoyed living in had grown enormously and was reflecting a value system we didn't want to raise our children in. Fortunately, Ed was offered a job in another area near a charming, small town. We moved in September 1981.

For us, the opportunity was not just good luck. Our religious faith had become more and more important to us as a family, and this move seemed an answer to our prayers. Also our faith had helped us all deal with Laura's diabetes. Despite the ten years of some perilous experiences, we were able to see it all in the context of life on earth as a series of trials and troubles. We did not question "Why?"—we accepted it as a part of a plan. Laura also benefited because of her faith: she did not see herself as a "bad" person being punished for a sin; she saw the diabetes as part of a special plan.

One major drawback with our move was that we had had to leave a trusted medical community behind. Without an endocrinologist in the small town, we finally found a physician who was aggressive in the management of diabetes. We had gone too far with Laura to leave her with someone who did not really know the disease very well. But we still missed our beloved endocrinologist Dr. Bejar!

Again, our prayers seemed to be answered. As our family grew up and with the ever present medical bills, I had found a secretarial job at the local university to assist with the home budget. One night after work while watching the news, I was surprised to see a professor from the school as part of a report on a diabetes care unit in a nearby city. He had gone to the unit for a complete examination and was sharing his very positive experience with the news media. A few days later, the professor and I shared diabetes experiences—his and Laura's. His enthusiasm for the diabetes care unit and its endocrinologist remained high. He recommended both for Laura.

Not too long after our conversation, Laura developed the flu.

Usually no big deal, the flu for someone with diabetes can be very complex. I talked with our family physician, put Laura to bed, and sat with her to monitor her sugar levels. At 1:00 A.M., I awoke to Laura's labored breathing and extremely high pulse rate. We called the doctor and took her to the local hospital.

Laura's blood sugar was 870 and heart pulse rate was 157 per minute! Her breathing was becoming increasingly more difficult; her kidneys were partially shut down! Deeply concerned, the doctor and nurses administered oxygen and large doses of insulin. Apparently with the vomiting and diarrhea from the flu, Laura had become dehydrated, causing her body chemicals to get out of balance.

Laura was close to death. I had never been more scared. They worked on my daughter for over three hours before admitting her to the intensive care unit. I prayed, preparing to accept what I could not yet understand.

Soon after her recovery and return home, I decided it was time to seethe diabetes specialist for a follow-up to the whole ordeal. We had the office visit in the city and admitted Laura to the hospital's diabetes care unit.

We were overwhelmed with what we saw and experienced. The entire hospital wing was devoted to diabetes care. The wing was casual, warm, and friendly. Patients could wear street clothes and walk around. A kitchen was provided and people were allowed free access to it for snacks. It even had a balcony with comfortable chairs so people could escape the hospital atmosphere if they wanted to.

The wing also had the latest in medical equipment. For example, Laura was hooked up to a computerized artificial pancreas. It drew blood, registered blood sugars, injected insulin as needed, and kept a record of everything. One could either monitor it all on a screen or review the computer printout later.

But the diabetes care unit did more than treat the disease. It also provided an extensive educational program. Every patient got a large teaching notebook. There were seminars, films, and a computer program that patients could use. Many of the medical staff were teachers. Frequently, they taught Laura on a one-to-one basis while treating her. The emphasis was on self-help and self-care.

Even an exercise bicycle was provided to emphasize the importance of exercise. The opportunity for exercise allowed patients to try to duplicate as much as possible a day similar to those at home with the usual activity, diet, and injections.

We were impressed also by the follow-up opportunities available through the diabetes care unit. A nurse truly committed to diabetes care called Laura about once a week to get her blood sugar readings, discuss insulin adjustments, and check up on her physical and emotional condition. A friendship rapidly developed, and Beth has become an important figure in Laura's life.

It has been over a year since Laura's visit to the diabetes care unit. Beth still calls, and I cannot convey what a blessing this has been—for Laura and for us as parents. She has taken from our shoulders sole responsibility for encouraging Laura to test her blood and to maintain proper diet control. Beth is a bridge who is so very welcomed.

So that is where we are. We have lived through much which has been emotionally draining for all of us as a family. Each person is affected when one member of the family lives with a disease such as diabetes. We all wonder: when will the next emergency arrive? when will we start seeing the complications brought about by a lifetime of diabetes? will we see the kidneys fail? the eyes? will we be faced with amputations or circulatory problems?

Certainly, the person who called diabetes the "silent killer" was right. To look at a young person with diabetes—like my Laura—from all outward appearances she looks vibrant and healthy. On the inside, who knows what is happening? I know all too well that at best insulin represents an imperfect solution to diabetes. Each person with diabetes has to live with that knowledge. So does each parent of a child who has diabetes.

Laura now is a freshman in college. She aspires to be a doctor. I admire her. She has set high goals in spite of the odds that she will face complications from her diabetes. She tries to live a life doing what most eighteen-year-olds enjoy doing. She does these things even though diabetes never lets her forget that she cannot have a completely "normal" life, as she is constantly reminded by the blood testing, injections, diet control, and insulin reactions.

I am encouraged by the diabetes research. I hold on to the dream of a cure one day very soon. God willing, someone will find a cure for this dreadful disease. But, until such a time, I continue to pray, thanking God for all things. And I continue to encourage Laura to do what the doctors advise her to do and to keep up her hopes for a bright future in spite of the seemingly insurmountable obstacles diabetes has inflicted upon her.

The Luck of Good Friends

RECENTLY WHILE IN the Philadelphia area, I took the opportunity to join three friends at the gaming tables in Atlantic City and to discover happily that my diabetes wasn't always mine alone.

Bruce, JD, Vince, and I had gone to the Sands' casino to play blackjack after dinner. In a few hours, we knew that we were "on a roll"—all four of us were winning! No matter who was dealing, we continued to win.

At ten o'clock, I glanced at my watch. It was time for me to check my blood sugar and take my evening injection. But I was winning. How could I get up from the table?

Bruce, JD, and Vince were aware of my recently increased involvement in controlling my diabetes. They had been observing my struggle with moving from one injection a day to two and finally to four—with the accompanying glucose monitoring.

"Time for your shot?"

Bruce had noticed my checking the time.

"Pretty soon," I muttered. The dealer had just hit my 13 with a 7 of diamonds—a winner.

"Let's go," said JD.

"Naw, we're winning. No sense ruining the karma. I'll do it later; I'm okay," I insisted.

"Well, we are leaving," Vince said, and they all gathered their piles of chips and started getting up from the table.

Hating to gamble alone, I had no recourse but to join them. We cashed in and returned to our hotel room.

I checked the blood sugar (120—must have been really relaxed), took my injection, and returned with them to the tables. The cards were cold, but that didn't bother me. I was too busy treasuring my increased awareness of what good friends I have.

My good fortune certainly extends way beyond a run of luck at the blackjack table. The support of friends—as well as loved ones—cannot be overestimated for any person—let alone someone with diabetes. Good friends are invaluable.

Meet the Endocrinologist: Marvin

He had wanted to be a doctor for as long as he can remember. From a rural background, he jokingly says "a doctor was the first person I saw who was not wearing bib overalls and that I 'imprinted' on him for this reason. . . . As a child I wanted to study nature and would have enjoyed being a biologist or a game warden or a forest ranger. I love the woods, and if I had not had a strong push from home to get an education, I could have gone into the woods. No one in my family had gone to college and my father had not finished high school. They knew what a doctor was, but had no idea that any one could earn a living 'studying nature' so becoming a biologist was not really something I ever considered."

From the age of four until nine, he suffered from pneumonia and had numerous occasions to visit the doctor. From this early, caring contact he developed a burning desire to be a doctor. Frequently attending a rural one-room community school, he skipped third grade and maintained the desire to be a doctor throughout junior and senior high school. Even in college the single-minded zeal for medical school was undaunted. He went to summer school so that he could graduate in three years. On occasion, he took courses at the same time from two different colleges in Pennsylvania. "I said in college that if I didn't get into medical school, there was no other vocation that I could possibly get into because my training was so pointed."

He started out to practice general medicine, but at medical school he developed an interest in internal medicine. "I discovered that I didn't like surgical procedures and didn't want to deliver babies, so the part of medicine left was internal medicine." While in the air force, he was assigned to work in an endocrine clinic and "found that I enjoyed this." That led to a fellowship in genetics, endocrinology, and metabolism. It wasn't until he was in private practice that he did extensive work with diabetes.

"I realized that caring for patients with diabetes brought together my previous interest in family practice in that I could deliver primary care to patients with a chronic illness and at the same time I could fulfill my desire to relate to the whole person."

ON THE JOB

On a typical day, he leaves home at 5:30 A.M., picks up his schedule at his office, and does rounds at two hospitals. Around 8:30 A.M., he returns to the office to see patients, to do administrative paperwork for the diabetes care units or the medical partnership, and to see non-medical appointments. If scheduled, he again sees patients. Mondays and Fridays frequently are split between patients and paperwork. On occasion, he must return to one of the hospitals for a consultation or to see one of his patients. Patients usually fill all of Tuesdays and Thursdays. Wednesdays—his "day off"—require that he do rounds at the hospital, go to his office to do more paperwork, and attend a variety of meetings. He tries to finish by noon. Every third weekend he is "on call," when he does rounds in the hospitals for all three doctors in the practice. He also answers any phone calls from patients throughout the weekend.

He views his history in diabetes care as a process of reflecting on, trying, and changing approaches to patient care. For this reason, he is absolutely certain that he would go into diabetes care if he were to start over again. In fact, his impetus would be to start more quickly and to change more rapidly in his approach to those with diabetes.

"In retrospect, I would have pushed harder for a 'unit' (a diabetes care unit) to be started years ago. Although in one way I feel like I am just now learning and now being able to put together some ideas that would make a unit valuable. I assume that five years from now I will be doing a number of things differently from the way I do them now, not that they will be 180 degrees different, but that I hope they will be far more sophisticated than they are presently. . . . I hope that we can be smarter about knowing what are the important aspects of patient care we need to emphasize in order to apply information properly."

The human side of diabetes provides both the joy and the pain of his vocation. The problem of application frustrates him as an endocrinologist. "The treatment for diabetes is 'simple.' Diabetes would be much easier to treat if it did not occur in human beings. . . . It also would be a whole lot less interesting to treat." The frustration comes from watching the disease progress in its ravages and from knowing that the real disease is locked away deep down inside of the patient. He feels the frustration of not being able to "get through" to patients so they will do what is necessary to handle the disease.

"I feel like I'm not really providing any service to these people and I struggle with trying to balance showing them acceptance and yet letting them know that I am unhappy that they aren't taking care of themselves properly. I see their failure as my failure and feel that I should be able to get through—some way. I feel that perhaps I'm too understanding of the excuses at times and at other times too insensitive to hear what the real problems are. I have a very empty feeling when patients like that walk out of the office, but usually I try to manage to be excited about their next office visit, thinking 'maybe next time I will say the right thing' or that circumstances will be right for getting them to apply the treatment necessary."

People with Type II diabetes who are chronically obese and who will not accept that there is a connection between the food that they eat and their body weight—and therefore the diabetes— perhaps most represent what frustrates him in diabetes care. "Some of these people have an incredible capacity to deny reality and what they are in effect doing is denying the single treatment that will be effective—that is to diet." He is frustrated by his inability to convince people to do what they know they should do.

This frustration, his as well as the patients', is why the endocrinologist wants more work done on the psychological evaluation of patients and their support structure. "Some non-cooperative behavior simply may be a reflection of anger at medicine in general, the 'system,' the physician's office, or the physician himself. . . . I would like to know where they are coming from. It would help to establish a healthy therapeutic doctor-patient relationship."

The joy of working with people with diabetes is "getting to know them and getting to share in the joys that they experience when they start to feel better about themselves because they are exercising, and have a certain degree of, control in their lives."

He holds a view that might not be popular with everyone. He

sees diabetes as an opportunity for personal growth. Sharing—if not assisting in—such growth contributes to his joy in diabetes care. "I think having a chronic disease like diabetes can be a great stimulus to personal maturity. In our present society, it is easy to escape and to blame external forces for the problems we all run into. We can change jobs, move, and change spouses and never be forced to admit that maybe the problem is not our employer, neighborhood, or spouse but ourselves. When one has diabetes, he cannot change diseases. He has the 'opportunity' to be forced to deal with a problem that is not going away."

THE PHYSICIAN'S ROLE

To this endocrinologist, the physician plays an essential role in helping the people with diabetes deal with their problem. He recognizes that the role can be demanding—if not seemingly contradictory. "First, I must establish a supportive, caring relationship which is meaningful to patients. They must know that I do, indeed, care about them as people and am willing to look beyond hemoglobin A1C values. Second, I must bring patients back to HA1C values and to act as a 'consumer advocate' for their eyes, blood vessels, kidneys, and so forth."

What characteristics does he think would help a physician fulfill such a role? He must be able to practice top quality, state-of-the-art medicine. That requires his keeping informed of the latest developments in medicine and medical treatment.

He must have an accurate picture of his capabilities and limitations, so that he knows what problems he is able to help his patients with and those that he needs to refer to someone else. This involves being a "team player." It involves turning to others who have abilities that the physician doesn't have but which are important for full diabetes patient care. As well as the physician, usually the team includes a dietician, a nurse educator, a social worker or psychiatric nurse or psychologist, and perhaps a community support group.

He must be able to listen, be intuitive, and truly care. "This has to do with accepting that the patient is more than just a patient, more than just a carrier of disease, but that he/she is in fact a person and as such has the right to be heard and the right to enough respect to have his own concerns seriously considered."

He isn't sure how to make it all work. He knows listening takes time and "time turns out to be the most valuable and most limited resource a physician has." He also knows listening requires attention to non-verbal as well as verbal communication. "The physician must listen with ears to the unconscious. He must hear not only the words, but he must be intuitive to be able to assess what the patient is really trying to say." To truly care for the patient, he recognizes that the physician has to be careful not to succumb to either his ego or his insecurities. It is too easy for a doctor to insist that he is the boss and that he is always rational, always smarter, and always right. For the doctor-patient relationship to have a chance, the physician cannot be "dogmatic" or "unapproachable."

He admits to having no answers to his own questions: How open should a physician be? How human should a physician be with patients looking for a god or for someone who has "the answers"? When is the patient's agenda as important as—if not more important than—the physician's agenda for treating the symptoms of a disease?

But he is unwilling to leave them unanswered or just to acknowledge his shortcomings. "I see myself as being very much 'in processing.' I'm learning how to create a team where the team not only maximizes my strengths and minimizes my weaknesses, but also feeds back to me those areas of weaknesses that I need to be working on. I want to enlarge the team. . . . I want to change my methods. . . . I want to continue to grow as a person. "

DEALING WITH PEOPLE WITH DIABETES

"I enjoy meeting newly-diagnosed patients in that I feel that I will be able to help them achieve an accurate perspective. I will not have to 'undo' bad habits. I simply have to work through misconceptions that patients may have from friends, acquaintances, or relatives. . . . Usually these patients are very motivated because they are frightened and because they have recently had symptoms. Working with them is usually fun . . . unless there is a lot of denial or if they have a lot of fears."

His goals for the patients achieving an "accurate perspective"? For those with Type I diabetes, the results are patients who check blood sugar on a regular basis, maintain a normal hemoglobin A1C, and proudly bring the homework of blood sugars to appointments. These patients are then able to modify insulin doses for meeting unusual circumstances in day-to-day living and to come to the physician for treatment of acute illness or complications. For those with Type II diabetes, the result is the acceptance of the connections between their weight and blood sugar and between eating habits and weight. Patients are then able to exercise personal control of their lives.

But to him the success of the right perspective is not merely acceptable blood sugar and HA1C numbers. "Successful" patients exhibit a great deal of cooperation, a personal maturity, and a willingness to try and to fail and to try again. He has had a lot of experience with those who for various reasons have been unable to be successful. "I usually do pretty well when I can remind myself that my responsibility is to inform and to try to push the right buttons to get them to turn around. My responsibility then ends and they ultimately carry the responsibility for their own actions." But he admits to being human—to getting angry occasionally or to withdrawing from those who "know it all."

He also has had experiences with uncooperative—if not abusive—patients. "My overall approach to people, whether they are patients or not, is to allow the force of whatever anger or abusive comments they have to dissipate by letting them get it out and listening to it. . . . My goal is to listen to these people, to explain when an explanation is called for, but not to try to justify myself. . . . The time when I have problems is if I am insecure and they, in fact, are pointing out something which in reality I am afraid to admit myself. If I have had no reason to be insecure—either personally or professionally—the abusiveness is not a major problem."

But he isn't always able to achieve objectivity and therefore to do what he would like with patients. "My feelings with a young child are primarily sadness. This is one situation in which I find myself being the least honest in that I feel that the situation calls for optimism more than it does honesty. . . . I guess the sad part is that, no matter how hard they try, they are going to have to face the diabetes and that, no matter how good a job they do, their life will still be different." With children of his own, he is very conscious of the burdens in just growing up. "I feel like children today have a very tough road at best, so it really hurts to see children who have the added burden of having a chronic illness which will require day-to-day 'work,' extra time, and extra expense." Part of the burden that he worries about are the complications. "I guess I look at them and my mind flashes thirty years ahead and I wonder whether we really are going to be able to prevent the complications with good control or what they are in fact going to be able to achieve with good enough control for these people."

In dealing with the human side in diabetes care, he seeks a balance between being too involved in the patient's distress and too professionally detached. "We are emotional creatures. We are human just like the patients are humans, and there is going to be an emotional interaction. I think this can be helpful. In fact, I think it is necessary, but it must be balanced."

OFF THE JOB

Despite the long list of responsibilities, the endocrinologist-unit director-business partner claims he has no problem at all in getting away.

He enjoys walks in the woods, target shooting, and photography. When he has time, he goes to the woods to camp and to hunt ("an excuse for camping"). He dreams of camping in Canada, British Columbia, and Alaska.

"This gives me a sense of perspective. Life comes and goes in the woods. I recall while hunting in Pennsylvania, I had come across some abandoned farmhouse and I can still recall the feeling of sitting there on a foundation of what once was a home, thinking about the family who lived there and thinking about those things that seemed important to them, the things that they spent their time worrying about, and now in fact, all of these things are gone and squirrels are running across the foundation of what was once their home, and I realize the same will be true for many of the things that are my 'concerns' from day to day, seeing the cycle of life moving on."

His sense of the transient nature of life may contribute to his persistent urge to write and his active work in his church. He keeps a daily journal of introspection, meditation, and prayer. Although he tries to read the Bible or a devotional book each morning, he wishes that he read more.

The center of his non-professional life is clearly his family. "I thoroughly enjoy the time with my family. I enjoy shooting rubber bands at my kids and getting them shot at me. I enjoy wrestling on the floor. I like sitting in the backyard on the back of a canal with my youngest daughter watching turtles, snakes, and birds. I am a playful person—verbal games, jesting, and teasing. . . . We have a lot of physical contact and our times together are often very light. We laugh at ourselves."

It is not surprising that his goals with his children resemble those for his patients. "My goal with my children has been to help them learn to 1) establish priorities, 2) be aware of some of their unconscious 'goings-on' and be able to express these in relationships with other people, and 3) gain problem-solving abilities."

But he knows that he is all too human, that on occasion he himself doesn't do what he asks of his patients and family.

"My life style may be described as 'not healthy.' The diet is fairly simple: cereal for breakfast, half the time I don't eat lunch or either I have a hamburger, supper is simple with no dessert—perhaps pudding or a half dozen cookies. My exercise regimen now involves primarily lifting weights and isometric exercising. I have had fits and starts on running on a trampoline, stationary bike riding. . . . I would hope to expand these."

He considers his failure to manage fully the stress in his life the greatest hazard to his health. He hopes to decrease the external stress "in the future," but now relies on his life view, journal writing, and humor to make his life "relatively healthy." He insists that he is in control of his life.

Having had cancer approximately ten years ago, this endocrinologist feels that he has a perspective which helps him empathize and therefore deal with others who have a chronic illness.

"There is obviously a limit to which I can empathize because I don't have the same problems as those with diabetes. I think I can empathize in part because I too have hurt. I too have been ill, and I too have faced the possibility of a serious disruption in my career and life plans. . . . In addition to personally having some of the same feelings, I have seen the effect of diabetes on people, families, spouses, and others. I can never say, however, 'I know how you feel' because I do not have diabetes."

From his perspectives as both doctor and patient, he firmly believes that the most ignored aspect of medicine is recognizing that diseases occur in people.

IN THE FUTURE

The endocrinologist is cautious about the future. He is afraid that too many involved with diabetes and diabetes care tend to "escape" present demands and difficulties by focusing on what might be. He prefers to point to past progress. Recent developments show the way for wrestling with the disease in the present rather than dreaming about when it will all go away.

"We are significantly more hopeful and more aggressive in the management of patients. We have home blood sugar monitoring, hemoglobin A1C's, newer insulins, and new injection techniques. We have tools and techniques to help normalize blood sugar and data which suggests that this is crucial. . . . These are tremendous advances, though they add significant pressure to patients with diabetes. Their target has been made smaller and therefore their work harder. The progress and data increase the demands of 'compliance' by narrowing the range of acceptable therapy and cooperation."

He expects that the future will build on such progress. He expects increased use of improved insulin pumps or similar devices, the disappearance of injections with syringes, better home glucose monitoring techniques, and further refinement of treatment goals and procedures.

A cure? "In ten to twenty years, maybe something that would be more readily defined as a 'cure' may happen. But, we may wind up not making the advances that we think in this area."

Professionally for himself, he foresees in five years more inpatient and out-patient diabetes care facilities actively involved in research. He hopes that they will include expanded and improved teaching programs to convey information, to train in treatment techniques, and to motivate patients with diabetes and their families. In ten years, he believes that the success in the treatment-teaching-counseling approach to diabetes care will have an impact upon the entire health care community in its care of the chronically ill.

Personally, in five years, he will be trying to get his children through college and planning for the days when that demand upon his resources will be over. In ten years, he expects to be reflecting more, spending more time in the woods, and spreading the word about the success he expects to document in the research surrounding the treatment-teaching-counseling approach to diabetes care.

After that he dreams of "backing off," writing, traveling, teaching, and giving more time to the other things he enjoys.

Finally, the endocrinologist-diabetes care unit director-partner-father-husband commented on his life: "It is kind of like piloting a boat. From time to time you get into water that is heavy enough that the primary thing you can do is to steer into the waves, even though they may take you a little bit farther away from where you ultimately want to be. I consider that frequently the water gets fairly heavy and I have had to steer into the waves. . . . I hope to do better than that."

Many a person with diabetes could probably say the very same thing about his or her life.

Meet the Diabetes Nurse Specialist: Beth

THE JOB

Mike: How many people with diabetes do you think you might have worked with?

Beth: In close follow-ups—where I help them monitor their blood sugars, assist with insulin doses, and just listen—I would say over 300. For short-term work without follow-ups, I've worked with more than 2,000 people with diabetes.

Mike: What are your primary responsibilities as a diabetes nurse specialist?

Beth: Since most of my work is done on a diabetes care unit in a hospital, I spent about 50 hours a week there. I am involved in doctors' patient rounds; insulin and oral agents adjustments; telephone follow-ups with patients formerly on the unit; one-to-one consultations with individual patients on the unit; group sessions with patients or nurses; meetings with primary care nurses, teaching nurses, physicians, and hospital administrators; program evaluation, development, and revision. Plus there is a lot of on-the-go question-and-answer discussions with patients, nurses, and physicians. I am a part of a diabetes care team. The team includes primary or bedside care nurses, two diabetes teaching nurses, the nurse manager, the clinical nutritionist, a diet technician, the head nurse, and the diabetes nurse specialist. But frequently—as with the other nurses on the team—I find myself a teaching-counseling-primary care nurse who does administrative work and who gives nutritional advice. I also attend diabetes support group meetings twice a month, but they are volunteer—not an official part of my job description.

Mike: What is the best part of treating and working with people with diabetes?

Beth: I love seeing them grow in self-care expertise, in hopefulness, in self-esteem, and in self-confidence. I enjoy their triumphs and victories in the trenches. I try to share the burden of the battle with them, particularly those with Type I diabetes. Type II diabetes is a different problem and usually requires more of a behavior modification approach in most instances than a cooperative sharing-the-burden approach. Type II requires the professional to wield authority, to dictate, to "punish." Such an approach is almost never appropriate, helpful, or effective in the setting of Type I diabetes—and it is unappealing and uncomfortable to me.

Mike: What is the worst part of dealing with people with Type I diabetes?

Beth: It's knowing that the task of maintaining sustained glycemic—blood sugar—control is incredibly difficult for the patient who, if at all conscientious, labors under the threat of unpleasant, dangerous long-term complications on the one hand and humiliating insulin reactions on the other. Such a host of factors affects and influences sugar levels, and many of them are out of the control of the patient and/or the professional.

The task is also difficult for the professional. The toughest part is knowing when and how to encourage increased vigilance and when and how to encourage a more relaxed stance. And I cannot discount the terrible impact that the complications have on me as well as the patient.

Also for me, the person with Type I who cannot or will not be honest, whose standard mode of coping is by manipulating people and distorting or misrepresenting facts, is most difficult. I'm not referring to the ordinary dishonesties with which people cover up—or try to cover up—their vulnerability; I'm referring to habitual, blatant, big-time lying in order to achieve one or more secondary objectives.

Mike: What is the worst part of dealing with people with Type II diabetes?

Beth: Type II is difficult to treat because it could be cured if the underlying eating disorder was controlled or cured, but that requires a behavior modification approach. Most people with Type II diabetes can have smooth glycemic control if and when they stick with their diets—which they have to think of as medicine—and avoid extra calories—which they have to think of as poison. In fact, when they lose about 10-20% of their total bodyweight, they often can get rid of their diabetes.

However, most people with Type II don't or can't do that so they have blood sugars in the 300s or higher all the time without symptoms. The result is that the long-term complications, especially retinopathy and neuropathy, start as early as five years after diagnosis. It is difficult to make any sort of effective connection with these folks without using very tough tactics.

Mike: What is the type of person with Type I diabetes who is easiest to work with?

Beth: The more open, up-front, and honest the person is the easier the person is to work with. But I would emphasize that the responsibility rests with the professional for making the patient-professional relationship one in which the patient feels safe and is able to trust the professional. The onus should be on the professional to practice the "therapeutic use of self."

Nevertheless, the person with Type I who seems to have the best fighting chance is one for whom the disease will be less of a disaster. Characteristics of the person with a better fighting chance in particular include 1) not getting the diabetes until adulthood—the later the better because of emotional as well as physical reasons; 2) possessing a very strong, robust sense of self-esteem and self-worth before getting the disease; 3) working from the beginning with a professional he or she trusts rather than fears; 4) having and enjoying a strong, close-knit support system not limited to the family; 5) demonstrating little need to be a perfectionist in areas of his or her life; 6) being intelligent, literate, and solvent; 7) possessing a strong sense of hopefulness; and 8) experiencing expert, compassionate diabetes care from diagnosis.

Mike: What is the type of person with Type II who is easiest to work with?

Beth: People with extra internal resources. They need them to accomplish the very difficult job of changing their eating behaviors, especially with those who are compulsive eaters. The resources or characteristics needed? People with Type II diabetes need 1) a strong sense of self-worth and self-esteem; 2) a strong, close-knit support system; 3) enough financial resources so that they are not worried about basic survival; and 4) a strong belief that the diabetes will cause severe harm if not controlled.

Mike: What do you think prevents people from being easy to work with?

Beth: Most people do the best they can. However, I do believe that some conditions exist that prevent people from doing well with their diabetes. First, they are subjected to health-care professionals who actually cause more harm than good, either because the professional doesn't care, doesn't know any better, or hasn't learned to communicate effectively. A second contributing factor can be significant others—family, friends, or loved ones—who demonstrate negligent or punitive attitudes or who are overzealous in their desire to help or to make everything all right. The third—and perhaps the most common—obstacle to effective treatment is denial of the diabetes. While denial has a valuable role in the coping strategies, it should be temporary as a stage or phase. If it becomes a constant, it becomes counter productive and a real danger.

THE RESPONSIBILITIES

Mike: What do you think is the diabetes nurse specialist's role or responsibilities?

Beth: I first must know what I am doing with the diabetes control regimens and work on learning more and more. I must be accessible without smothering the patients. If my knowledge or experience is insufficient, I must refer patients to other specialists. Also I should communicate—with the patient's permission—with the other members on the health-care team.

Second, I must foster a patient-professional relationship that is characterized by trust, hope, objectivity, honesty, and openness. These feelings foster comfort because patients don't feel alone with their justifiable terror. They also allow patients to express anger, pain, or grief if that is what they are experiencing. I should help the people with the diabetes feel that they are gaining a real measure of control over the disease and in their lives. I think this comes from the development of self-esteem and self-confidence as they become an expert in diabetes management. On my part, I have to be careful to treat the patients as adults—even if they aren't. I don't want the person with diabetes to feel indebted, more vulnerable, inadequate, insufficient, or "bad."

Mike: Do you think that a diabetes nurse specialist can determine patient behavior? If so, how?

Beth: Generally, people are responsible for their own behavior. However, in a therapeutic alliance, if the patient isn't doing well or is "behaving badly," I think we should look first at the professional and the dynamics and content of the interpersonal relationship. If this is done and the cause is something the nurse specialist cannot help, then the patient should be referred to someone else.

Mike: What can be looked into?

Beth: Foremost, does the nurse have the medical expertise for treating diabetes? Eager to learn more? Willing to continue the educational process?

Is the nurse willing and ready to listen to the person with diabetes as a person? Is the nurse sensitive to the person's feelings? Does the nurse offer empathy rather than sympathy? Have a sense of humor? Willing to share the burden? Able to put the patient at ease? Capable of accepting the patient as he or she is? Does the nurse have clear-headed, problem-solving skills? Can she anticipate trouble spots? Can the nurse set priorities? Identify and offer options? Effectively communicate? Can the nurse be persistent? Sense when to be gentle or tough? Compassionate? Aggressive or passive? Objective when advice is asked for?

Mike: What can a nurse specialist do to improve perceived shortcomings?

Beth: I "network." That is, I talk personally or over the telephone with other diabetes specialists and psychosocial experts about specific patient problems, recent medical developments, and their experiences. I also listen to the people with the disease. I consider them the real experts. Frequently they tell me about what works, does not work, and why.

I study—formally in course work and informally through reading the latest literature and attending professional conferences. I talk with a friend who is a psychiatrist about the personality traits of mine which could be threatening to the patients or to the therapeutic alliances I try to conduct.

THE RESPONSES

Mike: How do you feel when you meet a new patient who has just been diagnosed as having diabetes?

Beth: When I meet a new patient who has just been diagnosed as having Type II, I feel, "Thank goodness it isn't Type I. Let's get down to work on it." With Type I, I feel some sadness and some pain. To share some of the patient's distress is a normal nursing function. While feeling that, my first thought is something like

"Who is this person? What's the best way for us to get to work on this together? How can I be of help?" So the battle begins. The patient is no longer a solitary helpless victim. He or she now has people on his or her side to fight *with* them—not *for* them—along side.

If the patient is a young child, the diagnosis is really a catastrophe. The feelings are more distressing, but the work goes on. There are tears to share with the parents and with the patient if a pre-teen or teenager. Then comes the rage and terror and pain and grief—all rational, reasonable responses.

Mike: Do you ever get emotionally involved in a patient's medical problems?

Beth: How could I possibly participate in a real-life therapeutic alliance with a human being and not share his or her distress?

Mike: Do you believe a nurse should be objective when dealing with a patient?

Beth: I should be objective when dealing with data and events; I should be a human being when dealing with a human being who happens to be a patient. One dimension without the other is *worse than useless.*

Mike: What about detachment?

Beth: As a nurse, I shouldn't cling or be possessive. I should give the patient plenty of freedom to live his or her own life, to make his or her own decisions, to be his or her own person.

To be detached in the emotional sense—unmoved, untouched, unfeeling, being unwilling to share the patient's discomfort—is to remove the human dimension from the nurse. Such a nurse does actual harm by dehumanizing the patient, magnifying his distress, making his burden heavier, and isolating him with his terror, rage, pain, grief, and guilt.

It is absolutely necessary that my sharing in the patient's distress doesn't become something that is *my* personal distress. The most urgently needed thing to do with the felt distress is to allow it to be a positive force in the sense that the energy for working with the patient in a real therapeutic alliance is augmented.

Mike: How do you deal with a patient who has been ignoring your advice and is truly out of control?

Beth: First, I ask myself a number of questions. 1) Is the patient really ignoring me? Or did he not hear me? Did he forget what I said? Did he fail to hear or block out what I said? Was I clear or did he misunderstand? 2) What is really going on? Is he resorting to denial to such an extent that his safety—immediate as well as long term—is in jeopardy? 3) How can we together get at the source of the difficulty? 4) Is it time to decrease the frequency of contact? Is he afraid to say so because he worries that I will be disappointed or angry or something? 5) Is it time to refer him to someone else? To whom?

I always try the direct approach. I ask the patient what he believes the trouble is and if he has any suggestions for getting at it. For example, fairly recently, I had a teenage girl who was out of control and unwilling to deal directly with me. I tried everything I could think of and everything my consulting expert connections could suggest. Finally, I asked her if she wanted to work with another nurse. Her response was "Yes, I think so. I am mad at you about something you said a long time ago. I'm not going to tell what it is so it's no use for you to ask." So I referred her to the nurse she preferred. I wish that I had had more time to develop myself as a diabetes nurse specialist—but the teenager doesn't have all the time in the world for me to develop fully. I don't have unlimited resources and that distresses me. I, however, retain hopes that they will expand as I increase in age, experience, and knowledge.

Mike: Do you ever get frustrated, discouraged, or depressed when patients seem to ignore what you prescribe?

Beth: Sometimes I feel discouraged or depressed when patients seem not to benefit at all from the alleged therapeutic alliance with me. I don't blame the patient—the responsibility rests primarily with the medical professional.

The only thing that really makes me yell and scream is a persistent compulsion of patients to take too much insulin which defies reason, courts disaster, and makes your favorite daredevil look like a wimp. A large number of people I work with have this compulsion; naturally they are trying as hard as they can to prevent complications. The reflex insulin-dose-increase in reaction to a high blood glucose—without resort to reason—actually works against, not toward, the goal.

I recently have had several confrontations with a man about this after learning that his HA1C was less than 5% and that he had lost consciousness two times with blood glucoses of less than 20. Thankfully his wife was at his side and was able to administer glucagon. She told me about it. . . . When I attacked his autonomy by telling him that an HA1C less than 5% indicates frequent severe insulin reactions that are bad for him, that he needs to lower his insulin doses, and that I would be calling him in two to three days to hear about his dosage and blood sugars, he responded, "I wish to hell you people would get your stories straight. For years all we hear about is get that HA1C down. Now you're telling me mine is too low. I like it like that and I don't mind insulin reactions. If you think you want to call me again, you suit yourself." He was enraged. . . . But we have continued to work together. . . . I get so frustrated. I feel so ineffective. Life is hard enough without sorry excuses for the "help" we sometimes try to give.

Mike: Do patients ever get abusive?

Beth: Rarely. Once or twice I have been the target of flying objects. Once a patient told me to "get the hell out of here" immediately after I introduced myself and my purpose in speaking with him.

Generally, I give abusive patients plenty of time and space to settle down and reorganize themselves. It is important for them to save face. If the patient is always abusive or only abusive, I leave him or her alone. . . . Usually negotiations are reopened and work continues. That is always the goal—to keep working.

Mike: Do you do anything else which helps you deal with patients—cooperative or abusive?

Beth: I try not to take myself too seriously. I get into trouble if I lose perspective. I force myself to remember that what matters is how or what the patient feels. I am a servant, an assistant, a coworker.

The best way for me to retain perspective is to go on silent retreats. Nothing like a period of solitude for my putting myself in my place. When I am unable to get to an actual retreat, I find solitude and introspection working in my rose garden or going for a drive. . . . I enjoy reading, listening to music, walking in the woods, swimming in the ocean or a lake, and visiting close friends. I feel that such activities help to prevent my work with patients from turning into a battle of egos.

THE FUTURE

Mike: How would you describe the progress of treating diabetes since your involvement in treating the disease?

Beth: When I got into diabetes care in 1975, we were doing Clinitest and maybe two injections a day. We didn't know any better. We still don't know very much.

But I have seen the introduction of self-glucose monitoring and the concept of the patient as the manager of the diabetes care team in 1979. . . . The synthetic human insulins are a big improvement. Such changes encourage me.

Mike: Where do you think the treatment of diabetes will be in the next five to 10 years?

Beth: Ideally, diabetes care and diabetes education will become more human and more humane. I'd like to see diabetes care centers owned and managed by groups of people with diabetes. The emphasis and focus will be on the prevention of and coping with difficulties as human beings with diabetes.

In specific terms, in five years, I hope we will be able to guarantee that no complications will develop if blood glucose levels are maintained within certain parameters. I hope we will have clarified what blood sugar and HA1C levels are desired. I think—as an uninformed opinion—in five years that insulin will not be given by needle . . . perhaps nasal or rectal administration.

In 10-20 years, I think there will be a "cure" or at least a vaccine for Type I diabetes. If not that, then non-invasive blood glucose testing—there go the sore fingertips—and a closed-loop insulin pump which senses sugar levels and delivers insulin accurately.

Mike: How do you see diabetes? Those with the disease see it in gloom-and-doom terms; those without it seem to think it is just about cured—a condition that is essentially an inconvenience.

Beth: The gloom-and-doom attitude is more realistic than the disease-is-cured attitude. However, life goes on. The gloom is there underneath it or in the shadows because of the threatening doom.

But, if the person with diabetes can learn to use the tools or weapons available to lend some advantage in the struggle with diabetes and if the person has one or more trusted, competent allies on his or her side, that person can postpone the doom *significantly*. If the person with diabetes knows and believes this and continues actively engaged in the battle most of the time, then some of the gloom will be dispelled or at least lightened. The person who is working on the glycemic control is more hopeful than the person who can't or won't or just isn't.

Mike: What do you recommend?

Beth: To deny the gloom-and-doom is to force it to go underground where it wreaks havoc with the best efforts of the therapeutic alliance. It is desirable for the person with diabetes to express, to name his torment, to identify and expose feelings—terror, rage, grief, guilt.... To do so is to help relieve the emotional misery of having diabetes. The most ignored aspect of treating diabetes is the emotional or psychosocial aspect—the human side—of the health-care team as well as the patient.

Meet the Diabetes Teaching Nurse: Sandy

Sandy did not know throughout her childhood that she wanted to be a nurse. In fact, when people pressed her fora pronouncement of her career choice, she had said she wanted to be an accountant because of her love of numbers and her success in mathematics. Fortunately, she discovered that accountants "work alone" and that "you get bored." When she went to college, she chose nursing after strongly considering psychology, medicine, and pharmacy as well as accounting.

"I knew I needed a career that allowed me a lot of contact with people, flexibility, security, and somewhat medically-oriented. Nursing fit that for me."

She ended up in diabetes care almost by accident. Having interned in a burn intensive care unit and finding the "extended and intimate contact" with patients rewarding, she couldn't find a suitable burn unit nursing position. She became interested in diabetes care because of the teaching opportunities she discovered while working on a hospital floor that included those with diabetes.

"I wanted to specialize in an area of nursing that dealt with the psyche of the patient, not just the physical symptoms and treatment."

ON THE JOB

She hasn't regretted her decision to get involved in diabetes care and teaching. She didn't hesitate with her resounding "yes!" when asked if she would go into diabetes care if she were to start over.

Because she adjusts her schedule to the patients' needs, her job tasks are varied and do not fit into a precise order. Typically, these

270

tasks involve teaching people on the diabetes care unit how to live with their disease, evaluating the competencies of incoming patients, checking out departing patients to ensure that they have the information and the skills necessary for life after the hospital visit, doing follow-ups over the telephone with patients who are home, and meeting with medical sales representatives.

Obviously—as indicated by her job title—her primary responsibility is patient education. The teaching generally comes in two forms. On a typical day, she teaches a scheduled, organized class for inpatients, outpatients, and family members every afternoon. The majority of teaching, however, comes on a one-to-one basis. During the day, she teaches patients while assisting them with such things as glucose self-monitoring and insulin injections. She also is on call: when a patient asks for help or another medical team member sees that a patient needs more training, the diabetes teaching nurse is called in. Sometimes the best teaching occurs as she "visits" with patients and family members. Things come up which—when dealt with—can make the difference between effective and ineffective diabetes management.

Also, as the diabetes teaching nurse, she is called upon to do public programs outside of the hospital. An indication of her dedication is her volunteer work with a diabetes support group. The group meets at least once a month at night, and she serves as a facilitator for the group meeting. She helps guide the meetings, offers medical and personal advice, refers members of the group to others who may be able to provide some help, and listens.

THE PATIENTS AS PEOPLE

Her attitude toward her work is evident when she took exception to the usual term used to describe her position: diabetes educator. "I prefer to be called a 'diabetes teaching nurse.' I am, first of all, a nurse—not an educator. Also 'diabetes teaching nurse' sounds more like a mutual relationship. To me, 'diabetes educator' sounds like just something we *do* to a patient."

Her attitude involves much more than arguing the semantics of her job title. "The best part of my day is getting patients together— either in class or one-on-one and having it go well—a lot of talking and sharing together. The best part of working with people with diabetes is having the opportunity to help them lighten the burden a little—when they turn things around and really work on their diabetes and they like the differences they find in themselves and in their lives."

A central theme to this diabetes teaching nurse's approach is her relationship with the patients. "Diabetes can be a 'gloom and doom' disease! Anger, sadness, and depression are appropriate responses. My response to that is for the person with diabetes not to feel guilty for being mad or depressed or feeling 'the hell with it' occasionally. Sometimes it can be helpful for your diabetes teaching or counselor to take more responsibility occasionally to give the person with the disease a break temporarily." She firmly believes that patients should take the credit for turning things around. "How people choose to deal with and treat their diabetes is a personal decision at a specific time. It should be respected. People may change how they handle their diabetes at any time. I think people are their own doctors. The patient's relationship to *his* or *her* health-care team is instrumental in how they deal *his* or *her* diabetes."

Her response to someone with diabetes and a 'gloom and doom' attitude? "I try to communicate, 'Yes, you have diabetes. You didn't do anything to get it and it's really rotten you have it. I wish you didn't. But you do. What can you do about it constructively? After a while you have to let go of the anger and learn to live with the disease.'"

She thinks that the public impression that diabetes is cured is unfortunate. First, it is incorrect. Second, such an attitude until recently has prevented the focusing of public attention and therefore medical research on the disease. Third, that attitude can result in a person not getting the emotional support and understanding often needed in living with a chronic disease. Why does the public act as if diabetes is cured? She believes there are two reasons. "They are ignorant. They may not know—or realize they know—people with diabetes as it is an 'invisible' disease. They have absolutely no idea what people with diabetes live with. Second, they feel guilty. Diabetes stinks. We are limited in our tools for dealing with it. We feel powerless so we ignore or deny the existence of the disease itself."

Her role? "Any nurse working with patients should communicate a non-judgmental, respectful attitude. I don't have to agree with or condone their behavior or ideas, but I do have to let them know I respect their behavior as their choice. . . . As a teaching nurse working with people who are living with their diabetes 'ideally,' I try to communicate several things: 1) an acceptance of what they are doing by letting them know I won't reject them because of their coping limits with diabetes; 2) the correct, up-to-date techniques for diabetes care and *rationale* for using those techniques; 3) the information about the problems and complications of poorly controlled diabetes so a person can make an *informed choice*; 4) my willingness to share the burden of the disease with them and to love them; 5) my ability to offer ways to help them deal with the emotions—the frustrations, fears, and anger—that go along with diabetes. . . . I don't think any one person *determines* another's behavior. But I suppose that, for people with diabetes, we can influence or set a tone for how they view themselves and how they deal with their disease. I strive to be loving, positive, accepting, caring, listening, and informative."

Clearly, this diabetes teaching nurse isn't satisfied just to talk about listening and caring. Asserting "I need to be a better listener," she pursues this goal with a two-pronged attack. In a formal approach, she is working on a graduate degree in mental health counseling. She firmly believes that a strong need exists for all nurses—especially those working in diabetes care—to have a solid, strong background in psychology. In a little less structured approach, she takes every opportunity to enhance her listening and communication skills, to keep up-to-date by attending professional conferences and to read nursing medical journals, and to attend as many diabetes support group meetings as possible. She believes that such meetings help her most in trying to understand how people with diabetes feel and how they live with the disease.

The need for acceptance and other counseling skills for working with people with diabetes is apparent to the teaching nurse. She herself has very strong feelings about a disease she doesn't have. "Diabetes sucks. It demands the impossible from its victim— perfection. It naturally carries with the physical problems a host of emotional burdens—guilt, low self-esteem, a feeling of being sabotaged by one's own body. Diabetes—especially Type I—can be very unpredictable. It demands that the person consider its presence 24 hours a day in order to live 'normally' while trying not to dwell on its ramifications 24 hours a day. People who do cope and produce with some semblance of good control amaze me. You never get a break from it and that must be extremely difficult. I hate diabetes. The complications. Death. The pain, guilt, remorse, and grief that people with diabetes feel if long-term complications become a reality. My helplessness."

The most difficult patients for her to treat and to teach are those who share similar feelings. Perhaps that is why she is so intent on counseling skills. "Most difficult? Dealing with patients who are angry as hell and scared to death about their diabetes but are unable or don't feel safe enough to express these feelings. They are hostile and often destructive. I can understand, but it hurts me because I believe if they could open up and deal with their feelings outright it would be a little easier to live with their disease."

Dealing with the feelings of guilt and low self-esteem that people with diabetes frequently experience is, in her opinion, the most ignored aspect of treating diabetes. She is dismayed by the continued tendency to label patients. "I don't like the term 'non-compliance.' In the 1990s we still shouldn't be cataloging people as those who do and those who won't. People who are 'non-compliant' usually are knowledgeable in diabetes care. We need to concentrate on why it is difficult to follow a medical regimen and what makes it easier. How does a label help?" Personally, she even prefers the word "people" over "patients." Professionally, she follows up her personal feelings by preferring and enjoying the affective aspects of a person more than the medical/physical aspects of a patient. "In my job, I deal with the emotional domains a lot, which suits me. I love the people I get to meet. I really get to know the people well on a long-term basis. I like the fact that the actual relationship between the person with diabetes and the nurse is such an important facet of successful therapy. . . . I would make a terrible ICU (intensive care unit) nurse."

TEACHING NURSE AS A PERSON

While a diabetes teaching nurse, Sandy is first to admit that she would be all too human if she had diabetes. "I am sure I wouldn't always be a model patient. Diet would be the hardest for me. I fall off the wagon a lot now. I would feel guilty."

Her reactions to the people with diabetes are human. When she meets someone who just has been diagnosed as having diabetes, she admits to being "sad" and "overwhelmed." "But my sorrow doesn't control me. I am an optimist and I am hopeful. I believe they can have a future that is brighter than those whose diabetes was diagnosed 10 or 20 years ago. I try to stress the positive—a positive attitude for wellness—and to minimize the possibility of long-term complications. . . . When children are diagnosed, I have even greater difficulties. You can't expect children to live their lives in such a way—to deny things and to inflict pain—so they will avoid physical problems 10 to 20 years down the line. They cannot fathom that. I try to minimize the negative aspects and to encourage as much 'normalcy' as possible in their lives. It's hard. I really hurt for them."

What happens when people with diabetes she is working with ignore her advice and are out of control? "I feel sad, frustrated, discouraged, and depressed because every day I see the ramifications of poorly controlled diabetes. But I never feel guilty or that it is my fault someone ignores medical advice. . . . I don't know if that is good or not. Maybe I should feel more responsible. I just don't want to see the person or family suffer unnecessarily. . . . Yes, sometimes I get angry. Frustrated. Often I feel bad for the person because I honestly wonder sometimes how 'compliant' I would be."

What happens when patients get abusive? "I leave them alone if that is their urgent request. I offer my services to them, but I don't force myself upon them. . . . Again, it all comes back to the fact that they are people. It is up to them. It is their choice. I offer choices, reasons, and rationales—not just instructions. I try to listen to what people say and respect their needs and limits. Whether treating or teaching, I want to individualize the health care. I want to share the burden with them. I try to help people feel safe—that I'm not going to chastise or criticize or dislike them. Honesty is important to me. I try to help them believe the importance of good control. I find out what motivates them. But I make it clear that the way they handle their diabetes is their choice and I will respect that. I will be available if they like."

How does she keep going—keep dealing with the chronically ill every day? "I see a lot of people who are working hard on getting well and staying there. That makes me feel good."

OFF THE JOB

Another way Sandy avoids professional "burn-out" is by playing hard on her time off. "I can relax with friends. None of them are in the medical profession so I don't talk about work. We have fun and laugh a lot." What does she do for fun? "My favorite thing to do when I am alone is to listen to music. I also read a lot. Rarely watch television. Never write. I am on a volleyball team—which I love—and we play once a week and drink beer and go out to eat. I *love* to eat out or over at a friend's house. (I don't love to cook.)....I have a wonderful, varied circle of friends, some I get together and party and dance with. There are others who I have a more quiet time with—talking mostly. It depends on what we need at the time."

When not on the job as a diabetes teaching nurse, she is active in an experimental theater group, a local woman's group involved in social issues, and a neighborhood association which is attempting to save the residential character of her part of the city.

When asked about her life style, she was candid. "My diet is not consistent. I go through months of eating in a healthy manner, followed by a period of falling off the wagon, and eating just what I enjoy. My meal times are sporadic. I love breads and protein. I like fruits and tolerate vegetables. I enjoy drinking alcohol—moderately —usually.... I get exercise although I do not have a specific plan.... I don't smoke or use drugs.... I consider myself healthy. I live spontaneously. I generally keep late hours. I love to sleep in.... I think changing my eating habits would be the best thing I can do for myself."

She proudly she sees herself as someone who is in control of her life. "Yes... I always felt that I could do anything with my life that I decided to do."

IN THE FUTURE

Her visions of the future in diabetes care are relatively specific. She hopes that in five years home glucose monitoring will be universal for all people with diabetes, human insulin (insulin genetically engineered to more like natural human insulin and therefore will not generate antibodies that will resist its effectiveness) will be more prevalent, and that more support for the team approach—endocrinologist, nurse, nutritionist, counselor—will exist. She suspects that more treatment and education of people with diabetes will take place on an outpatient basis and that hospitalization will be the last resort.

She expects in ten years that islet-cell transplants will become a reality, most people will be using smaller insulin pumps and glucose monitors, and that blood sugar monitoring will no longer require piercing the fingers.

In 20 years, "a cure! And I gladly will find another realm of nursing and counseling to work in."

Her visions for her own future are not as specific. With an M.A. in counseling, she hopes in five years to be in private practice with other diabetes care professionals and as a consultant to area endocrinologists. "I would love to work helping people with diabetes cope with the disease. I would like to work part-time with patients in the private practice and to teach part time at a university." She would like also to publish a book about diabetes from the health team's perspective, speak at medical conventions, and "become rich and famous." Then she would earn a Ph.D. and travel for pleasure.

LAST REQUEST

"How about a questionnaire for people with diabetes asking them what they need, expect, and want from their health-care providers and what they hate about their health-care providers?"

Support Groups:
A Prescription for Loneliness

Diabetes can be a lonely disease. Unless another member of our immediate family also has the disease, we can feel that we are the only person in the world wrestling with the disease. As we follow our diet, take our insulin, and sweat through our exercise, we can feel that we are alone. We begin to believe that only we experience the fears of having a life-long, chronic disease. Intellectually, we know that millions of people have diabetes, but emotionally it seems we are suffering alone. Suffering alone compounds the suffering.

One solution for suffering alone with diabetes is diabetes support groups. In diabetes support groups, people with diabetes, loved ones of those who have diabetes, interested parties, and health-care professionals get together to share information and experiences, to learn from each other, and to enjoy each other.

As with any solution, the diabetes support group may not be for everyone. Frequently, it just depends on the support group's goals and/or on the chemistry of the people involved.

For some, a support group offers a community of people who happen to have diabetes and who are willing to help each other out in whatever way possible. Regardless of the get-together's program, theme, or occasion, members of the group can talk about diabetes in general or their own particular experiences. If they wish, they may focus on the "down" side of having diabetes: they can talk about catastrophes, complications, losses, and deprivation. At Christmas parties, they may moan over how Christmas used to be "before diabetes got them." When the discussion is about food, it can turn to restrictive diets or grotesque comparisons between what they can eat and what "normal" people enjoy. A program designed to focus upon what the members of the group can do sometimes turns into testimonials that begin with statements such as "before I got neuropathy, I used to enjoy. . ." or "I enjoyed bicycle riding un-til I became so afraid of insulin reactions" or "I love food most of all. . . ." Other times history dominates: histories of bad doctors, histories of crippling complications, histories of people who did not take care of themselves and who lived forever, and histories of those who practiced rigid control and went down the tubes in no time flat.

But, most people who have diabetes are sensitive to the pitfalls when talking about the disease they have in common. Members of support groups can focus on what they can do, what good has hap-pened in their lives, and histories that have turned around for them. They also may be sympathetic to those who are suffering physically or emotionally. Specific advice, tentative suggestions, and possible sources of help can become the common fare of a give-and-take support group.

Such a support group serves its members in a number of ways. For some, it provides a safety valve for their anger and despair. They feel they can say what they want because that is one of the primary opportunities offered by such a group. Also, it provides an audience of others who may have felt the same way. For others, the group provides an identity. The meetings of a group which has something in common gives the members a sense of place within a world so ready to label them as "abnormal" or "different." As a re-sult, they focus on what is their common denominator—diabetes. A few may attend because they are in emotional pain. A diabetes support group shows participants that they haven't been singled out for diabetes. It allows them to feel that they aren't being punished, that they aren't evil, that they haven't been damned. Such meet-ings also may give people a chance to remind themselves that they are human, are doing the best that they can, and that they aren't the only ones who "slip up" with their self-care. But mostly they show people with diabetes that they are not alone.

But not all support groups have (or have to have) a helpful give-and-take chemistry. Many people find comfort in a social support group.

These support group meetings get together only for fun. All meetings are parties. The group provides an atmosphere which al-lows people to "let their hair down." Since they either have diabetes or are very familiar with what it is to live with the disease, they have the appropriate social graces for a support group that is primarily social. No one asks, "Is that on your diet?" No one counts the calories. (Usually, the food doesn't demand a calculator to keep track of the total.) Rarely are doctors, injections, insulin reactions, or toes mentioned. People in the group have picnics with menus that may even include beer and hot dogs; they ride horses and go on hay rides on a ranch; they swim and water ski at the lake. They may celebrate special holidays or the third Thursday of the month. The agenda may differ, but the goal is always the same—having fun. Diabetes is only a common denominator for creating a guest list.

But again the social support group may not be "what the doctor ordered" for some people with diabetes. Many might prefer an out-patient support group.

The out-patient support group is upbeat and educational. Frequently, this group is an unofficial extension of a hospital or a doctor's office. Generally, it is run directly or indirectly by health-care professionals who volunteer their time and energy. People with diabetes come to the group meetings to learn more about diabetes and to obtain advice about their own particular battle with the disease. Along with the acceptable refreshments, there are formal and informal presentations by doctors, nurses, nutritionists, and representatives of the local chapter of the American Diabetes Association or the Juvenile Diabetes Foundation. Over fresh vegetables and sugar-free soft drinks, diets are exchanged, blood sugars are compared, exercise programs are examined, progress reports on current research are given, and announcements are made. The group acts like a task force making war upon diabetes: always forward, never backward; upward and onward. Information is backed up with encouragement.

Of course, not all support groups have a single personality. Furthermore, there are more than three types of support groups. Many support groups may have mixed purposes. One group could be composed of the give-and-take, the social, and the outpatient personalities in a variety of proportions. A person with diabetes usually can find whatever concoction best suits his or her needs.

Then there are always individuals with diabetes like myself. I am not comfortable in any diabetes support group, regardless of the chemistry. Perhaps, I am more into denial than I have admitted, or I really haven't come out of the closet with my diabetes. It may be a "pride thing": "I don't need any help!" Nevertheless, for years, I essentially have preferred to be alone with my diabetes. But it isn't a desire to suffer alone. (I don't enjoy suffering at all or being alone very long.)

In fact, upon reflection, such resistance to support groups sounds silly—if not stupid and immature. (I'm very big into name-calling when an indefensible stance is exposed.) I keep saying "diabetes support groups aren't for me," but I am unable to dig up any convincing reasons. Comments like "they depress me" or "I don't have the time" don't exactly have an authentic ring to them. Especially when sometimes I do feel lonely—very lonely—with my diabetes.

But that's my choice and is something I need to work out for myself. For others, however, support group can be a powerful cure—a miracle prescription for loneliness as well as improved diabetes management. A wide majority of participants have found them to be, at the very least, worthwhile experiences.

The important point, it seems to me, is to know that a variety of diabetes support groups exists. Another is to remember that we have choices: we can choose the kind of group which is best for us or we can decide not to participate in one at all. However, even *I* recommend that anyone trying to deal with diabetes should give support groups a try.

What The Experts Would Do

WHEN SEEKING ADVICE, I frequently ask the experts what they would do if they were in my circumstances. I ask the repairman whether he would fix my old water pump or replace it. I ask the guidance counselor at my son's school if she would enroll her daughter in that program. I ask my friend if he were going to buy a new fishing reel which one he would buy. While certainly not fool-proof, I have found that this method of inquiry provides answers—whether verbal or nonverbal—that can help me decide what to do about the pump, the school program, and the fishing reel.

Why not use this same method for evaluating my diabetes management system?

I asked an endocrinologist, a diabetes nurse specialist, a diabetes teaching nurse, and a clinical nutritionist two questions: If you had Type I diabetes, what would you do to treat yourself? If you had Type II diabetes, what would you do to treat yourself?

The following represents their answers. These answers reflect what they would do given their particular age, life style, philosophy of life, personal preferences, and medical histories. Each cautioned me that what he or she would do might not be appropriate for someone with different circumstances. Therefore, the following is offered to indicate the preferences of four members of my health-care team.

TYPE I DIABETES

Endocrinologist: "I would use an insulin pump, human insulin, and would check my blood sugars two to four times a day. I would stay on a diet such as I am now on although I would be sure to eat three meals a day and eliminate the simple sugars. I would try to increase my cardiovascular exercise to 30 minutes a day. I would check my urine for protein at least three or four times a year and do a creatinine clearance test (for kidney function) at least once a year. I would get exercise electrocardiograms once a year. What I am saying is that I would be 'compliant.' I hope that I would. I think honestly that I would be, but you never know."

Diabetes Nurse Specialist: "Personally, I would take four shots a day of Regular and Lente human insulin. I would take the Regular before food and the Lente at bedtime. I would not use an insulin pump. I would probably try to follow a high fiber diet, but would not do well with it because I am not used to thinking about what I eat that much. I'd probably only walk for exercise.

I would try hard not to let the regimen make me work less. I'd certainly not be an ideal patient. I'd be more fearful of insulin reactions than complications. I am forty already. Losing consciousness or control of my actions would terrify me, so I'd probably let my sugars run high."

Diabetes Teaching Nurse: "Diet would definitely be the hardest factor for me. I'd fall off the wagon a lot. I would *try* to work out with a nutritionist a 1200-1500 calorie diet that minimized vegetables and red meat, maximized breads, and allowed for Lite beers several times a week. I would try to bike or walk daily. I would continue with my volleyball and dancing for fun. Biking daily would be realistic because I enjoy it a lot.

I really think I would do the blood glucose monitoring, via the Accu-Chek three to four times a day. I would take two to three days off per week. I would have to be on a pump (Eugly) or multiple injections because of my life style. My mealtimes can vary greatly and I love to sleep in late on days off. The dilemma is that injections hurt (I take SQ allergy shots twice a week), so it would be depressing sticking myself four times a day. The alternative, the pump, would still be a little hard to hide in my clothing as I live in shorts and t-shirts. I would probably opt for injections.

Another problem with the pump is I am not sure if my support person, my husband, could ever feel comfortable checking my blood glucose, shutting off my pump, and administering glucagon if I am comatose or convulsing one night. He is petrified of physicians, hospitals, etc., and I know my having diabetes would bring unbearable stress into our marriage.

I would probably end up binging and feeling guilty a lot if I had diabetes. That is, I *already* binge and feel guilty, but the ramifications of doing this with diabetes are horrifying.

Knowing what I do now, I would see an endocrinologist and follow with a diabetes nurse specialist and use human insulin. I would definitely need to see a counselor on a regular basis. I would be very angry."

Clinical Nutritionist: "I would take insulin in as many injections as possible to control my blood glucose. Probably it would be Regular before each meal to give me the most flexibility. I am not sure of the pump, but I would consider it. I would follow a high fiber diet since I do now. I would run and do aerobics for exercise."

Type II Diabetes

Endocrinologist: "I hope I would be scared into losing weight and get involved with an exercise program."

Diabetes Nurse Specialist: "With Type II diabetes, there is not much choice. There is nothing to do but to practically quit eating, walk more, and take pills."

Diabetes Educator: "I would monitor my blood glucose two to three times per day, five days a week. I would still try to exercise. Obviously, the biggest problem would be dieting which is *vital* in controlling Type II diabetes. I would try the three-day fast and core diet first to try to lose weight quickly. I would attend Weight Watchers—as I do now—to help long term with my battle with dieting."

Clinical Nutritionist: "I would lose weight!"

Appointments:
Why Every Three Months?

As I approached the doctor's office, I could hardly breathe. It was time for my regular three-month appointment.

I was early so I decided to walk down the street in an attempt to calm my pounding heart, aching lungs, and shattered nerves. The walk helped some. I faked a calm exterior as I entered the office.

I was lucky for this appointment: it was one of the first in the morning. Few people were in the main waiting room. I signed in, sat down, and cracked open a novel. I had to wait only fifteen minutes: this was one for the record book.

Calling "Michael," the nurse ushered me into the station for a check of vital signs. She wrote 160/100 for blood pressure. I was surprised: three blood pressure checks at home over the last two weeks had ranged from 130/80 to 140/86. My pulse rate was as atypical. It was 77; earlier checks of my pulse had been revealed rates between 56 and 60 beats per minute. After checking my weight (up three pounds) and height (down one inch?), the nurse moved me into an interior waiting room. I returned to the novel.

I was called to the small laboratory for a blood drawing. Back to the waiting room and the novel.

Several chapters later, I was escorted to a small examining room. The novel was left untouched as it occurred to me that my journey from waiting room to nurse's station to the laboratory to the waiting room and finally to the examining room reminded me of my visits to a crowded Walt Disney World. (At Disney World, management arranges waiting lines so that they wind back and forth but remain within close proximity of the desired attraction. The attraction's organizers instruct their personnel to keep smiling and to keep the winding lines moving. In these ways, they can disguise that the public frequently is waiting for a long time.)

"Hello."

The diabetes nurse specialist swept into the tiny examining room holding the medical file.

"How are you doing?"

"Fine," I lied. My anxiety over the appointment and my irritation over my recognition of the Disney World waiting scheme provided a curious emotional mix that I felt throughout my body.

"Well," she continued, "your blood sugar was high—365."

I cringed at what I perceived to be her arched eyebrows. She didn't seem to notice, but my response to her perceived reaction startled me. I thought that my knee-jerk response of guilt and self-loathing had been put behind me. I had thought that I was firm in my confidence that I had been doing the right things and that the guilt was no longer a part of my diabetes. My glucose test strip had shown a clear-cut 240 that morning, hadn't it? I had taken more than sufficient insulin (four extra units), hadn't I? Hadn't I eaten only an English muffin for breakfast?

As the nurse asked questions and took notes, my mind raced searching for some explanation as to how I had messed up. Somehow I mustered answers to her questions until she retreated from the room with assurances that the doctor would be right with me.

The novel held little interest as I waited.

But come the doctor did. He swept into the small examining room with a huge smile on his face.

"How are we doing? I understand you're having some problems."

The doctor chatted for several minutes with me about high fasting sugars, chest pains, and the possible need for laser treatment in my left eye. I did most of the talking—about the symptoms and about what I thought were the causes of the symptoms. The doctor briefly examined me with his stethoscope, thumped me a few times, and moved toward the door.

"You seem to have a pretty good grip of what is going on. It seems to be that you might be a prime candidate for an insulin pump. You might want to talk with some pump users about their experiences."

I became extremely self-conscious about my symptoms as well as my catalog of physical and emotional explanations. I felt pretty silly about my complaints.

"Okay," I replied, "but you know I have little confidence in machines. Plus I really would find it difficult to forget that I have diabetes with a pump strapped to me."

"Well, think about it. . . . See you in three months. . . . I'll have the nurse recheck your blood pressure. . . . Good bye."

With forms in hand, I headed for the accounts window and then the appointment window thinking about this three-month regular appointment. I recalled the sequence of emotions: the fear . . . then the manipulation . . . the guilt . . . the self-doubt . . . the frustration . . . the feelings of silliness and self-consciousness. It all seemed pretty aggravating.

Then I thought of my other three-month appointments. Overall, they didn't seem to have been much different than this one. Unless a medical emergency had existed, few of them had seemed very worthwhile. I began to question why I had been making these regular three-month appointments. Then I wondered why I kept the appointments. They did not seem to accomplish much more than create extreme anxiety, elevate blood sugars, and bring back ancient feelings of guilt and failure. Besides the usual blow to my bank balance, the cost of the appointment seemed too high.

This particular appointment's costs were all too common. A severe headache had developed. A wave of exhaustion had engulfed me as I had walked out into the sunlight. A total sense of despair hung over me.

Rationally, I could understand why the doctor wanted me to keep regular three-month appointments. Patients can report symptoms and ask questions about their treatment program. The early detection of complications can lead to effective treatment which can prevent permanent damage. New discoveries from recent research can be passed on. Lab tests can track the relative success of current therapeutic programs. Adjustments can be recommended.

Emotionally, however, the need to keep tabs on my condition and current research seem to be outweighed by what I experience as an ordeal. If I have worked hard trying to manage my diabetes, I feel that it isn't good enough. It never seems to be; something could always be better. Even those who have managed to maintain excellent control (How do they do it?) may discover that the stress of the appointment may distort findings which seem to contradict records of controlled sugars and regular blood pressures. Even those who maintain excellent control will take extra doses of insulin and eat less than their prescribed diet before an appointment in efforts to insure a "good report card."

If I have slipped up with my diet or exercise or medication—and who doesn't?—I feel like I have betrayed the doctor, the nurses, and myself. Also I am sure that they will find me out and either indirectly or directly chastise me for my "noncompliance." I am certain that behind their furrowed brows run thoughts that I must be stupid, weak, dishonest, or suicidal. Again unusual efforts are devised to disguise such previous indiscretions.

Also with the regular appointment comes the terrible anticipation of the bad news that has been long promised to anyone with diabetes. Will it be this visit that reveals problems with the eyes, the heart, or the kidneys? What will the treatment involve? What specialist will I have to see? What piece of modern medical equipment must I confront and tangle with? What will be the physical, emotional, and financial costs involved in fighting whatever complication is setting in?

Regular appointments with a doctor? Every three months? Rationally they make sense, but emotionally they are at best an ordeal. It is no mystery why so many who have diabetes either don't make regular appointments or don't keep the appointments they do make.

Perhaps both parties might reconsider the whole terrain of regular appointments. I might try to remember how much an emotional reaction can interfere with the vital functions of seeing people who are professionally trained for treating the disease. To help ensure that the appointments accomplish their vital functions, I should strive not to see myself as an opponent of the health-care professionals. Doctors and patients are not supposed to be enemies, but a team. Symptoms and problems should not be concealed. Inaccurate impressions should not be created for the appointments.

The tasks of the health-care professionals are as difficult. Whether the doctor, the nurses, the nutritionist, or the lab technician, they should try not to allow long hours, repeated histories of noncompliance, and patients' troublesome emotional conditions to result—on their part—in uncaring attitudes, despair, and burnout. They can be seen as angry parental figures, prison guards, and wrathful gods who seek to punish transgressors. The appointments should not turn into ineffective mechanical routines.

The physician and I need to ask ourselves, "Why every three months?" and to come up with answers that focus on wellness, teamwork, honesty, respect, sensitivity, and understanding.

The Physician's Response to "Appointments: Why Every Three Months?" by Marvin C. Mengel, M. D.

As I look at today's schedule—hospital rounds, office patients, consultations, and oh so many meetings—my mind tiptoes quietly, so quietly that I can hardly hear.

It looks hectic today. . . . It looks like I'll be late for lunch. Lunch? Hah! Well, at least that time will give me the opportunity to catch up. Maybe I'll be on time with my first patients of the morning. . . . It looks like I won't get those extra dictations done today . . . and the phone calls. I really don't like to return phone calls. At least I won't have the time or opportunity to think about them until later this afternoon. Maybe some will take care of themselves. . . . At least I don't have to think about them now. After all, if someone is sick, we would have told him or her over the phone to come to the office. . . . Phone calls. Those dreaded phone calls are explanations of late lab work, telling bad news to a family, or announcing unwanted news of unexpected pregnancies. . . . I never seem to get the chance to give good news—just varying degrees of bad news. Boy, how would it be to pick up the phone, hear the bated breath, and say "Everything is wonderful!" That would be great . . . to hear the breath sweep out into joy!

Back to the schedule. . . . I hope I have some people who are easy, no major problems. . . . I am tired today. I sure do not feel like deep thinking. Would an easy day of miracle healing be too much to ask? . . . Enough. I need to remember when I was a kid and went to the doctor. The conclusion of the visit was so important. "What did the doctor say?" I'd be asked when I got home. The verdict. It seemed then there needed to be a verdict each time. I needed to have something to carry home with me—some new treatment, some new hope, some reassurance of immortality. . . . Now the shoe is on the other foot. What can I give? What will my patients carry home? What will they say when their family asks, "What did the doctor say?". . . . I need to remember to give them something. . . . I forget sometimes, but I try to remember.

I'd better get started. If I fall behind this early in the morning, I'll be an hour behind by lunch. . . . I hate that.

Into room 5. . . . It's Mike: intelligent, "reformed," takes his care seriously. He has turned around so quickly and so well that I kind of hate to see him. . . . I am afraid I'll mess it up. . . . What can I give him today?. . . I don't know. His sugar is high . . . so is his blood pressure. . . . Bad news surely is not going to reward him for all the good work. . . . Well, he didn't seem too delighted with those suggestions. Maybe I've made a mistake making those suggestions. . . . But then, he's the one who is upsetting himself. I should be able to show him that I can make a few simple suggestions that will help his control. That should encourage him. . . . No way. Look at that face. . . . I couldn't do any better myself. In fact, I realize that I probably wouldn't do as well.

I need to keep moving.

I messed up with Mike. . . . I started by talking about a lab result—a measurement. That sure isn't human. I do that when I am in a hurry. . . . How about a little "human talk"? Talking with people is more fun than talking about blood sugars, especially since I really don't have anything to offer. . . . I know Mike has had some chest pain. . . . I didn't need to have started my day that way. . . . Chest pain. He certainly is a candidate for angina. . . . Anything I suggest is going to cost money. I'll need to twist his arm. . . . I know. I'd be the same way. . . . Cardiologists are just plain expensive. . . . He has had such negative experiences with doctors anyway. . . . It really doesn't sound like angina, but it sure could be. . . . There's no way to win. If he sees a cardiologist and it is not angina, he'll be angry about the cost. If I don't have him see one and it is angina, I could do him a lot of harm. If he sees one and it is angina, I'll feel better—I got it right and he didn't waste his money, but he'll feel worse. . . . Why, oh why, did he have to have chest pain today? It sure doesn't help my efficiency this early in the day. . . . Well, I do not think it is angina. I'll wait.

I should see him sooner for his next appointment. It makes me nervous to wait three months. If the pain goes away though, I'd rather wait six months. . . . I'm not sure I gave him anything today, but one of these days I will, so I need to keep seeing him. I need to keep facing my own failures, my own uncertainty. . . . Deep down I believe that I am doing him some good. Having to see me helps him to take better care of himself in between appointments. In fact, I'd rather see him every month for that benefit, but then the cost *would* be too much. . . . How often should I see him? How often should I see the rest of my patients? Every three months.

A pat on the back, a touch, a farewell. . . . Did I really give him anything? A reason to come back?

I've got one thing to be thankful for: I don't hand him the bill. That would be tough. Did I give him something worth X amount of dollars?. . . . Oh, rationally I know I am no more expensive than someone less "specialized." I am no more expensive than his family practitioner. I am at the right level for charges. . . but I am glad I'm not the one collecting the money. . . . Part of me wants to be "nice"—to make him like me by giving him a discount. I know better. I fight the urge every appointment. . . . I am a professional—just like he is—and this is a fair charge. . . just don't ask me to collect it.

Regular appointments? I have no problem with people who have Type II diabetes—if they have lost weight like I have encouraged them to, asked them to do, threatened them to do, begged them to do. Their blood sugars would get better, and their visits would become far less frequent. In fact, most of the Type IIs would be "cured" and would hardly ever have to come back. . . . I don't have any problem asking these people to come back every month if need be because, on one level at least, they have a choice.

It's the people with Type I diabetes I have trouble with. No matter how hard they try, they should never get out of the routine and the need for a regular visit. . . . I'd like to give them a longer time between visits—six months, a year, whatever—yet whenever I do, I regret it. . . . What's magical about three months? Nothing. Why not four months? An as-needed basis? There needs to be contact.

If I care and if I am involved, I must give them a time to come back. When I was a doctor in the military where the medical care is free, if I told the patient to come back when he or she feels the need to, some people would come back within a few days. Others would deny symptoms and never come back. If I give patients a time for a follow-up appointment, they find security in a designated time period. Sometimes transient symptoms that occasioned immediate returns by the military patients go away by the time a patient returns for a regularly scheduled appointment. If the symptoms are severe, they will come in early, but otherwise they tend to wait until their appointment.

How long is too long? I don't know. But three to four months is too long without contact. . . . Perhaps a phone call—oh, I hate phone calls!—in between would be helpful. Some find it necessary. Others need a gentle reminder to keep follow-up appointments.

The financial cost—too much . . . but not if I can help prevent or delay open-heart surgery or kidney dialysis. The only way for me to live with the cost is to see it as an investment. . . . I not only feel that way, but also rationally believe it . . . especially when I go from one examining room to another to find patients who have lost their vision or have had open-heart surgery or a serious foot infection.

Every three months? You bet!. . . . I can understand Mike's failures. I can understand the cheesecake. I can understand his slipping from the rigid adherence to a difficult schedule. I am human too . . . But the heart and the kidneys don't understand. Someone has to be an advocate for them. Someone has to say—no matter how valid the reason—if your blood sugar is over 300 for eight hours or four hours or maybe two hours or maybe less, something inside your body is getting hurt. . . . I need to be human and understanding because if I am not I may get in the patient's way as he tries to do the best he can. To do that would be disastrous. But, I must balance the understanding with the real world. "Understanding" does not prevent the damage of a high hemoglobin A1C. "Understanding" and "good reasons" are no match for the harm that continually elevated blood sugars do.

I try so hard to walk that thin line between my natural rigidity and my sense of acceptance and knowledge that I would do no better. But I cannot forget all that I have seen.

Every three months? Not if he bores me with normal hemoglobin A1C's, a record of stable retinopathy, an absence of chest pain, no encroachment of neuropathy or infections, and an endless string of normal blood sugars. Bore me with that data, free me from my terror for you, and do that for two or three regular three-month appointments—then I'll think about every four months or five or six. But bring me elevated blood sugars, abnormal A1C's, high blood pressure, advancing neuropathy, or increased frequency of chest pain, and I'll feel like three months isn't enough. Regular appointments every three months haven't prevented things. I need to see you more.

Go ahead, complain about money. I would too. That one always gets to me. I feel guilty because I have a nice home, a nice car, and an income more than I ever dreamed I would have. . . . I feel even more guilty because he is a teacher. If I felt he was overpaid, it would be easier. . . . I can't win there either. . . . But, if my regular intervention delays or prevents his disability, it seems more than worth it to me. But, as he must feel about students who leave his class, I will never know—I will never know if I was responsible for a success. . . . Catastrophes are another story. If you have one or more of those, both of us will feel I should have been able to prevent each of them. We will feel that you have been cheated. At least I will.

Every three months? You bet.

I'm behind. I spent too much time. . . . I'm not sure I really help any more for the time I spent. . . . I'm leaving Mike feeling a bit uneasy. Things are unfinished. I feel less "successful" this visit. . . . I sure hope that I have not been too heavy-handed. . . . Maybe I was too easy. . . . I sure hope I haven't gotten in his way. I don't want to reverse the progress that he has made. I just want him to have the best chances that he can.

Into Room 4 . . . a patient with a goiter. The thyroid was underactive last time. Now it is up to normal. The nurse reports that the patient is feeling much better. . . . What a break! What a pleasant break! A person who feels better, who tells me she is glad she's here, who doesn't mind paying me because she got what she came for, who is doing so well. I can say, "Come back and see me in a year."

I walk out feeling better. I have accomplished something. The patient is better. Having done something lifts my spirits. . . . I'm ready with renewed strength to move ahead to my next patient with diabetes. . . . I am quietly thankful for patients with thyroid disease.

Walking toward Room 3, I am interrupted by my nurse. There is a final question from the previous patient. She has asked, "Why every year? Why can't I just get my thyroid prescription filled? Why do I have to come back every year?"

Teaching Toward Compliance:
A Patient's Perspective

WHY IS "NONCOMPLIANCE" so widespread among people with diabetes? Why are young and old, male and female, black and white, Type I's and Type II's, sixth graders and Ph.D.'s, day laborers and attorneys not taking advantage of all that diabetes educators have to offer?

It seems to me, as a classic noncompliant and as a teacher, that major keys for improving patient compliance involve how the diabetes education occurs.

I know how it feels to have the disease, to be subjected to the well-meaning instruction, and to be reminded—oh so frequently—how important strict control is. As a teacher I also have experienced the frustrations that one can have when he offers information, solutions, and help only to have it ignored—if not thrown back into his face. Ah, the thankless pain of caring about a group, of knowing what they should know, of trying to convince them of its importance, and of having all of the efforts essentially ignored!

In 1955, I left one of the world's foremost clinics for diabetes destined to be a classic noncompliant. I had learned that diabetes is a disease of impending disasters. The entire educational program was characterized by threats. Each lesson began with the menacing assurance that such and such disaster would happen to me if I did not do whatever was prescribed exactly as directed.

Every lesson rigidly demanded perfection. Inquiries about possible deviations from the prescribed regimen were met with less than subtle and sensitive resistance: "Everything you eat that is not on your diet or in the ordered portions will shorten your life." That one's work, studies, or play might not conform to a rigid schedule would not be considered. The person with diabetes who wanted to have a chance of living would have to adjust. The demands for rigidity had dominated every lesson, every prescription for survival, every encounter with the medical profession, every experience with my family. The instructions and reminders about every ramification in having diabetes had been persistent and insistent orders for perfection.

Thus, beginning as a child, I had found it easier just to deny that I had the disease. Imperfect, guilty, and doomed, I had "reasoned" that I should enjoy myself as best as I could for as long as I could. I was going to pretend to be normal until I had to join those who were blind, lame, or dead. "Compliance"? Why bother? Diabetes is a bloody, painful, expensive disease which constantly reminded me that I was mortal.

As an adult—despite my education, experience, and seeming maturity—I suffered with despair surrounding my diabetes and with the urge for denial and therefore noncompliance. Now I don't.

This dramatic change began with an educational experience on a modern diabetes care unit. As a teacher, I learned a great deal about teaching. As a person with diabetes, I started to free myself from my past prisons and to develop a means for my compliance. Perhaps professional diabetes educators may benefit from my personal experience by considering the following suggestions.

First, remember to treat the patient as a person first and a person with diabetes second. Nothing disturbs me more when dealing with physicians than their looking up from my medical records and saying, "So you're diabetic." Right away I feel myself pigeonholed as the monolithic "diabetic" to be treated as all others with diabetes who have passed through the office with the "usual" symptoms, problems, and dismal future. The appearances of relying upon formulaic responses not only can undercut the effectiveness of any therapeutic program but also result in an adversarious relationship with the patient. I have no difficulty recalling sequences that went like the following: "So you're diabetic. What seems to be bothering you? How have your sugars been running? How much insulin are you taking? (I am briefly examined.) You know you should be careful about such and such. Stick to that diet. Keep those sugars down. Let's run some lab tests. Make an appointment to see me in about three months."

Although the diabetes educator's prescriptions may be absolutely correct, too often they become a litany that is always repeated, is always the same, and always comes out sounding like a recording played for each patient. Unless the diabetes educator looks at me and sees someone with a low self-concept because he has diabetes, a Type-A personality, a father of two young sons, a fierce competitor, and a pointy-headed intellectual who would doubt his own mother, little opportunity exists for an alliance in combating diabetes.

Too often we find themselves reading materials for people with medical degrees or for someone with only a third-grade education or watching filmstrips on foot care with talking socks as the stars. By knowing and recognizing who the patient is, the diabetes educator can tell what would be appropriate. To approach patients with information that they may already know, with pre-fab treatment programs, or with programs too sophisticated to be educationally effective can sabotage any efforts to help the patient. The psychological effects can be far-reaching. To neglect to adapt to the patient is to invite a "who cares?" attitude. Without the patient's wholehearted and sustained participation in the therapeutic alliance, hopes for effective education and treatment are futile.

For example, during my first experience, I was a "juvenile diabetic" or the "juvenile diabetic in ward 410." A few months ago, I was Mike, an English teacher, a father of two young sons, or a clown with silly tee shirts—who happened to have diabetes. It wasn't just semantics. My treatment and my education were for Mike, not for any or all people with diabetes. Linda, the clinical nutritionist, and I built my 1800 calorie diet with a high fiber and vegetarian slant—she did not just hand me a printed sheet of exchanges as so many others have with their stern admonitions to follow it. She created my diet after an extensive interview with me about my teaching, consulting, and tennis schedules; my food preferences and eating habits; my desire to gain or lose weight. She responded to my circumstances by educating me about diets and by offering two diets that I might use. My current diet is the first one that I have stayed with because it is the first one I helped make and therefore wanted to follow.

Second, let us know we are not alone. While trying to ensure that the patients are treated as individuals, the diabetes educators also should remind them that millions of people with diabetes exist and have been through the same experiences. While our cases are particular, we are not the only victims out there. The outreach programs, support groups, and individual counseling by others with diabetes can prove to be invaluable resources that the medical profession can turn to for assistance in relieving the emotional stress in dealing with diabetes.

During one effective teaching session on the diabetes unit, Sandy, the diabetes educator, neither lectured nor showed video productions; she let the patients talk. It came as a shock to me that so many very pleasant people also happened to have diabetes. Surely they weren't being punished for anything; perhaps I too just happened to have diabetes. They had been afraid, angry, and despondent about diabetes and had gone on to take up their own fight against it; perhaps I too could hope to progress beyond denial and noncompliance. Some patients confessed backsliding and non-compliance; perhaps I too could work toward reclamation without fears of accusations or character assassination.

Third, present the education and the treatment as a positive action for wellness we sense we can choose. Effective teachers ask students what they wish to accomplish and offer a number of possible ways for accomplishing the chosen goals. Telling people what not to do doesn't usually work. Diabetes is by nature a restricting disease that begs for rebellion: "Don't eat this" and "don't drink that" just provide a shopping list for noncompliance. Positive suggestions to "Eat combinations of more complex carbohydrates such as dried beans and rice for reduced insulin dosages and fruit for energy" give people a sense of having some control over their lives.

Give something to work for rather than against. Gaining rather than not losing sounds more worthwhile. It may seem mere semantics, but most would prefer to save their eyes or limbs rather than not lose them. I don't think that threats work. Just about every health-care professional who has treated me has threatened me. Oh, it was always polite and in my best interest, but, make no mistake, a shortened life and a hellish life of complications are threats. I went to the diabetes care unit because a nurse convinced me that I could help myself.

Success consciousness is common sense and effective psychology. Encourage rather than find fault. Success breeds success; failure leads to despair. Anyone can find flaws in anything, let alone diabetes treatment. Control always can be tighter. Rewards or warm fuzzies for small gains can generate enthusiasm for greater compliance and more gains. Diabetes is ripe with bad news; a little good news can go a long way.

For years I avoided blood sugars for fear of the justly deserved abuse that they would occasion. Rarely was I disappointed. While on the diabetes care unit and since I have been home doing my own glucose testing, no blood sugar report has evoked even a hint of accusation or judgment. Low ones are applauded; high ones only elicit recommendations for insulin adjustments.

This encouragement led not only to regular testing but also to better control. After a few weeks of testing, I saw that the two shots daily were not effective. Beth, the diabetes educator who was following my progress, told me that some take four shots a day or go to an insulin pump for better control. She never ever said that I *must* or *should* try something different than the two shots. But the results from glucose monitoring were clear to me. I chose the opportunity to give myself four blood tests and four shots a day. This is someone they take kicking and screaming to a doctor and who passes out just driving through a hospital zone! For twenty-eight years I had resented taking one shot and never had had my blood sugar tested. This remarkable change came because a diabetes educator *introduced* me to what was available, *gave* me a sense that I could make changes if I chose to, and *encouraged* me in whatever choice I made.

Fourth, remind patients that diabetes educators are human. For years I had seen doctors and nurses as deities who have all the answers. As a result, I tended to relinquish responsibilities to them for my health care. When something went wrong or did not work, it was their fault. Much like composition students who would prefer to explain their deficiencies by pointing to the unreasonable demands of the instructor, people with diabetes frequently allow the health-care professionals—who don't have diabetes—to serve as absolute authorities who therefore make unreasonable demands that only gods could live up to.

However, when the health-care professionals remind me that they are human and therefore neither omniscient nor omnipotent, I do not entertain unrealistic expectations for them. I can see myself as a valuable part of a team for treating me. I can be an active participant rather than a passive agent in the process. Gods would not need me.

Also, as humans, health-care professionals are not expected to know everything: they can say "I don't know" and won't see the patient pass out in shock. They can involve the patient in the information- gathering process. With a history of honesty, when they do speak or advise, they will increase the chances of not only being listened to but also followed. Perfect gods who know it all easily become adversaries who are worshipped but ignored. For either students in an English class or people with diabetes, it is easier to be honest and open with a human, to admit failings and feelings, to present the full picture in the writing of a failing composition or in the weaknesses of a treatment program. Whether learning to deal with diabetes or how to write, people must recognize that each is an imperfect science that can and must be worked on by humans.

Fifth, try to prevent patients from becoming cripples entirely dependent upon the diabetes educator for treatment, motivation, and support. Certainly, be sure to explain *why* patients should learn how to take care of themselves, to show them *how* to take care of themselves, and allow them to demonstrate and to *practice* what they have learned. But, do not neglect to insist that they take primary responsibility for their own care. Diabetes educators serve neither themselves nor the patients well if they become a crutch which the patients come to depend upon entirely.

When I left the diabetes care unit, I went home with more than a fighting chance to be successful. While on the unit, I was expected to assume more and more responsibilities for my own care as each day passed. By the time I checked out, I knew what I should do, how I should do it, and that I had been doing it correctly. What a sense of power and independence! What an impetus for maintaining the habits of testing the glucose, adjusting the insulin, watching the diet, and feeling some semblance of control! The unit's staff provided me the opportunity for developing self-respect. I did not feel like a pet on a leash who had to turn to my owners every time I needed something.

Sixth, try to get patients to establish a dispassionate, objective attitude toward treatment. The horrible by-product of my early experiences came with my emotional involvement in my diabetes. My self-concept vacillated inversely to my blood sugar levels: the higher the sugar, the lower the opinion. When complications set in, I assumed I was being punished. I felt guilty about having a disease that set me apart, cost money, demanded special attention, and threatened my family's well-being.

Then, well-meaning health-care professionals—while working in the best interest of the patients—either threatened me with the evils of side effects, reproached me for real or imagined acts of noncompliance, or cheered me warmly for good results. To me, the messages sometimes seemed unclear, confusing, and distressing. Frequently I found myself torn between my desire to please others and my need to be me. The diabetes educator-patient relationship can add complicating dimensions to an already complex emotional environment. The guilt-and-denial cycle worsened as I failed to measure up to desired standards. I could not face the disappointments caused by my failures. Who could make rational decisions in such an emotional framework?

An objective, problem-solving approach to diabetes can avoid the stick-and-carrot, punishment-reward emotional spiral and the pitfalls inherent in dealing with human beings. If I am not afraid of disappointing my doctor, nurse, diabetes educator, or wife and therefore of having to face their pain and/or rage, I can then move beyond the emotional complexities and focus more on the treatment of my disease. Thus, diabetes becomes an enemy rather than a slippery terrain for maintaining personal relationships.

Seventh, remember that diabetes is a bloody, expensive disease. Sometimes state-of-the-art treatment can be seen too easily as financial overkill. Certainly, the expenses maybe necessary. However, I can recall the doctor ordering an office glucose test just an hour after lunch when I had done my own test. On another occasion, I was talked into buying a microprocessor glucose monitor. For several hundred dollars, not only was it expensive but also difficult to use. Upon telling the recommending physician, he admitted having never used the machine: he had seen advertisements for it. With two sons with enormous appetites, I found myself harboring some resentment. Incidents such as these provide all sorts of rationalizations for denial, diabetes educator-as-adversary thinking, and noncompliance. Although not very bright, it is an emotional reality for us.

Eighth, be accessible. While you cannot be expected to function as diabetes outreach or support groups, diabetes educators can create a sense of accessibility that can create more wellness and compliance. For example, recently I developed an infection in one of my toes. Rather than ignoring it, I called my doctor's office and talked with a nurse about the toe and what might be done. I have avoided a "situation" because I believed that I could call and make inquiries. On the basis of earlier experiences with these health care professionals, I did not feel that I was invading their domains, making a nuisance of myself, or being a crybaby.

While some danger of abuse exists, the establishment of accessibility can open the communication lines between the patient and the people trying to help treat him and, in turn, can help keep problems from getting out of hand. It is tough treating a patient who won't trust you, talk to you, or tell you how he or she is really doing. This trust and openness comes from trust and openness.

Thus—as someone who has diabetes and is a patient, a student, and a teacher—I would suggest to diabetes educators that one way for improving the success rate for combating noncompliance is to allow themselves to listen to and to learn from the patient. Even the pathological noncompliant may have something to offer that can help in treating and educating others with diabetes.

Teaching People to Learn How to Live with Diabetes: A Checklist

ALL HEALTH-CARE providers are educators. Those in diabetes care especially are under tremendous pressures to be effective teachers. How many teaching methods are there and what methods are available to diabetes educators? The overwhelming news is that for every educator who seeks to teach there is a teaching method. The challenge in that news is that any teaching method that exists may be appropriate for diabetes educators. An entire discipline exists to help diabetes educators be more effective teachers and to raise their consciousness of themselves as professional educators.

In the search for more effective teaching, health-care providers need to know that there is no one right way to teach. There have been several hundred studies comparing one teaching method to another, and the overwhelming portion of these studies shows few if any differences between approaches. The evidence to date gives no encouragement to those who would hope that we have identified a single, reliable, multipurpose teaching strategy that we can use with confidence that it is the best approach.

Likewise, all the scientific and medical information in the world about diabetes, in my opinion, will not insure patient adherence to treatment programs. To me, to increase the degree of adherence, health-care providers might consider the following suggestions:

1. Try to see yourselves as diabetes educators as well as doctors, nurses, nutritionists, or whatever;

2. Try to remember that the treatment of diabetes involves much more than information and procedures;

3. Try to recall that the delivery systems—formal and informal—for bringing information to a student-patient can be as im-

portant to the effectiveness of the treatment as the treatment itself is;

4. Recognize that a veritable cornucopia of teaching methods exists to assist you in achieving your educational objectives and seek them;

5. Adopt and use a set of criteria for evaluating specific teaching methods in order to insure that the particular method fits you, your student-patients, your objectives, and the contexts of your teaching situation;

6. Strive to help create an ideal curriculum for your student-patients—whether from a hospital unit, an out patient clinic, or a doctor's office—that starts with the vital information, moves to information processing, integrates social interaction, and culminates with increasing human awareness. In fact, I would not even insist on such an order, only that the human side of the educational models be included.

As a teacher, I am committed to such approaches to any educational situation. Today, every educator should try to help students not only to learn the basics, but also to develop the capacities for applying the basics and for adapting to conditions in the "real world" that often are less than "typical" or"normal."

With this attitude—if not these particular teaching approaches—health-care providers and therefore diabetes educators can make differences that will effect the lives of people with diabetes for a lifetime. They can defuse a lot of patient explosions and a great deal more pain.

When to Change
Health-Care Professionals

AFTER ATTEMPTING TO establish a therapeutic alliance with a health-care professional, sometimes people with diabetes—or any "patient" for that matter—find they are uncomfortable or unhappy or dissatisfied with the doctor, the nurse, nutritionist, or hospital they have chosen. Sometimes they cannot put their finger on what it is, but for some reason they wish they were free of that choice.

Unfortunately, if you are at all like me, "cutting" that member from the health-care team is very difficult—if not nearly impossible to do. I am a coward. I don't want to hurt anyone's feelings. Perhaps, I need some sort of assertiveness training because, no matter how dismayed I am with that particular medical professional, I cannot bring myself to sever the relationship and to seek out a replacement with whom I might be more comfortable.

I come up with all sorts of rationalizations for not doing the dirty work. I find myself saying things like, "They know more than I do. They are the expert. How dare I contemplate that there might be someone better out there? Who am I to question them?" Along the same lines, I tend to rationalize that "they are the best there is so why bother looking around?" Or "if I go to another replacement the whole process of giving a medical history, of the preliminary lab work and examination will have to be done, and we will have to spend forever getting to know each other. . . . Plus finding someone who has an opening!. . . I might as well stay put and save the hassle."

Then I always want to give them a second chance. Appointment after appointment, I leave muttering, "This is the last time I am going to put up with that sort of treatment!" But put up with it I do. Or "that didn't really happen. It must be in my imagination. I must be too sensitive; no one—let alone a medical professional—would say those things to me. Silly me." Or "I expect too much.

Here I am assuming that I have important concerns or serious questions or grave anxieties. I should have more faith."

This catalog of rationalizations is a mere sampling of the sorts of things that I come up with so I won't change doctors or replace someone on the health-care team. I have had more than my share of experiences where I felt that I really should "juggle the line-up" of my health-care team or at least send some of them "down to the minors." But I never had the guts to do it.

To my mind, having the opportunity to cut a member of the professional health-care team is essential for the effectiveness of a therapeutic alliance. Most important, it seems to me, is to maintain confidence in all the members on the health-care team. I need to feel that I have the best available on my team. This way I can have confidence in what is prescribed or recommended. I can feel safe. Furthermore, I need to feel that each member of the team is *my choice*. If all of them are on the team—and remain on the team—because I want them to be there, it seems more likely that I will participate in the therapeutic alliance. If it's my team, I'll probably play. If I choose the team, I'll want my team to win. In contrast, if I am unhappy or uncomfortable with a team member who remains on the team because I don't have the courage to make a trade, I may just avoid that member. Or I may just unconsciously set out to "prove" that my instincts or judgment is correct—by sabotaging the treatment. I know that isn't very bright, but being too chicken to assert myself can turn me into a strange quagmire of emotions and actions. All too quickly the "offending" person can become a scapegoat for the diabetes treatment not going well. That person—rather than the bozo who hasn't exercised, who has overeaten, or who has allowed stress to drive his sugars up—takes all the blame. This "opportunity" to blame another inhibits the chances for me to examine what I am doing and then making the necessary changes. Also one can use up all his energy being angry at the team member—and himself for not doing anything—and have little left for sustaining an effective treatment program.

Now I have come up with a way to handle the rationalizations and thereby go through with cutting someone from my health-care team. The following is a checklist of indiscretions, mistakes, or abuses that health-team members have been know to commit. I use this list to keep track of what is going on between my health-care team members and myself. Each time that I feel an indiscretion, a mistake, or an abuse occurs I put a check next to the item. I try not to use the list as a set of accusations, but as a means for graphing the terrain of our relationship. By keeping an actual checklist, I have a concrete record of what I felt has happened. I am able to evaluate the quality of our therapeutic alliance and have something that does not fade under the pressure of cowardice and rationalizations.

As the checklist darkens with amounting tabulation of seeming transgressions, I begin to evaluate the respective therapeutic alliance. If the "evidence" becomes such that it cannot be ignored—no matter how badly my knees are shaking—I have a record that can help me talk with the team member in question and, if need be, have something substantial that I can use to steel myself for cutting that team member.

The following represents my checklist of possible occasions for having a heart-to-heart talk with a member of my health-care team or for changing a team member. The listing is not in any particular order: no single item is meant to be weighted any more than any other, although I am always concerned about how up-to-date their knowledge of diabetes is.

Occasions for Change

When they threaten you, they seem like the enemy, or they frighten you.

When they won't consider the chance that they may have made a mistake.

When they are absolutely certain about how to treat diabetes.

When they lie to you.

When they do not listen to you.

When they will not admit that they did not hear you or did not understand you.

When they do not give you the chance to ask questions.

When they do not have the time to explain or are unwilling to explain a treatment, a laboratory test, or a drug.

When they do not examine you thoroughly during a medical appointment.

When you have to refresh their memories of your medical history.

When they say you are lucky to have only diabetes or that it could be worse.

When they treat only your diabetes.

When they focus on only one facet of treatment for diabetes, such as insulin or diet or exercise or medication while ignoring the others.

When they do not offer a choice of treatments.

When they prescribe a treatment regimen without asking about how you have to lead your life or how you would like to lead your life.

When they do not stress the importance of diabetes self-care.

When they do not present diabetes treatment as a positive act for wellness.

When the progress of your diabetes represents a threat or a boost to their ego.

When their knowledge of diabetes and diabetes care is out of date: some indicators might include ignorance of blood glucose self-monitoring, of the existence of insulin pumps, of the new insulins, of hemoglobin A1C tests, of high fiber diets, of the danger of exercising when blood sugars are high, of the new research concerning the causes for diabetes, of area or regional diabetes specialists and diabetes care units, of useful current reading materials on dealing with diabetes.

When they decline to inquire about obvious strategies that you use to "explain" unhealthy blood sugars and elevated hemoglobin A1C results, to avoid follow-up appointments, or to ignore your diabetes.

When they insist that you only use a certain specific pharmacy, laboratory, or hospital without providing a concrete reason.

When outside interests are more important or receive more attention than the practice of medicine.

PART V

All the Difference

What's the Good News?

A FREQUENTLY REPEATED test of how people see life is to ask them to describe a glass of water that is half-filled (or half-empty). Those who describe it as half-filled are seen as optimistic; those who describe it as half-empty are thought to be pessimistic.

Perhaps certain people with diabetes, doctors, nurses, and family members should consider taking this test before dealing with diabetes and people who have the disease. How these people perceive water glasses, diabetes, and life can influence others' perceptions—to say nothing about their own outlooks. A positive attitude towards life in general and diabetes in particular by those who deal with the disease can serve to create directly or indirectly a similar attitude in those trying to live with the disease. Such an attitude, in turn, can foster a positive approach toward the disease as a problem-solving procedure for wellness.

In contrast, if those who work with diabetes assume a "half-empty" attitude, they may pass it directly or indirectly onto others who are approaching water glasses, diabetes, and life. They are allowed to assume or they learn that there isn't enough water, that diabetes is the enemy, and that life is to be endured (or isn't worth enduring). Everything seems like a desert—without an oasis; like combat—without hopes of winning; like a dark experience—without a light.

The importance of attitude and therefore approach can be crucial. Consider, for example, the following actual demonstration of the effects of attitude upon me.

After nearly three decades (1955-1983) of insulin-dependent diabetes, I decided I should see just where I stood medically. During the extensive medical work-up in the hospital, I thought I had been through every medical test possible. The seemingly endless list of tests included such items as blood work, urine work, x-rays, a heart echo test, an eye examination, and an urological work-up. I left the

311

hospital shaken and with a new diabetes regimen, but thankful that it hadn't been worse. I went home determined to fight for the best life possible.

Months later, while at a support group picnic with Judy, Eric, and Bryan, I happened to come upon an old friend, a high school classmate's father. Joe, the friend in his sixties, had contracted Type II diabetes sixteen years earlier. However, the meeting of the friends was not entirely fortunate. Diabetes dominated the conversation during what was meant to be a family outing. Joe was suffering with severe neuropathy: he could not feel his legs from the knees down and hence shuffled when trying to move about. Joe was bitter and angry when he talked with me.

I was upset when I returned home with my family. I was thinking of Joe and then of my own diabetes. As each day passed, I became more and more distraught about Joe, diabetes, and my own future. Eric and Bryan started asking Dad, "Are you okay?" "I am fine" did little to reassure them. They sensed that I was getting depressed. They were certain, however, that I was not being as careful with my diet, glucose monitoring, and exercise routine as I had been before the picnic. Tentative about my treatment and uncommunicative in general, I was harboring doubts. I was afraid that I was losing the battle to Enemy Diabetes and worried about how close I was to Joe's state. Feeling increasingly hopeless, I was prepared to surrender.

Joe wasn't to blame.

As my attitude worsened and my attention to my treatment program slipped, Beth—a friend and diabetes nurse specialist—asked me what was wrong. "Nothing" led to "not much" and then to the story about Joe and finally to the whole catalog of fears. A discussion of complications, of the reported value of control, of current research, and of diabetes as a "bad news" disease followed. Beth kept trying to assure me that Joe's history was not mine and that Joe's problems need not be mine. I was skeptical. Predicting the future rarely provides a convincing argument for hope.

But Beth was undaunted. She looked through my medical records, especially those from the latest work-up. She discovered two bits of information. First, the neurological work-up showed that I had better-than-normal nerve responses in my legs and arms. In fact, probably as a result of a life-long commitment to exercise, my nerves were in great shape. Second, lab reports showed that I enjoyed relatively unimpaired kidney functions. She provided the hard data to convince me of the good news.

The results of this information were astonishing. What good news! Two of my greatest fears over complications were calmed. I was encouraged. I began to smile; the depression lifted; I began to have hope again. I returned to my aggressive approach to my diabetes by monitoring my blood glucose, following my diet, exercising regularly, and adjusting my insulin. I started talking about diabetes again. Judy, Eric, and Bryan were delighted to have a happy father back with them.

This dark period of personal suffering—and resulting lack of control—might need not have happened. If I had heard this good news while I was having my check-up and experiencing significant changes in my life and my medical treatment, I might have been able to resist the depression that the encounter with Joe had occasioned. Certainly, the health-care professionals and I had intended my hospital stay as an opportunity to evaluate my medical condition and to improve my treatment program. Unfortunately, the desire to correct problems too often overshadows the good news. Bad news gets the attention. Things that are wrong call upon the expertise of the doctors, nurses, and nutritionists. They naturally focus on what needs to be healed, cured, or corrected.

Nevertheless, I ought to have known that my nerves and kidneys were in good shape. Such good news—the knowledge that two major parts of my body were working—could have provided the will to work for more good news even when confronted with possibly distracting or distressing tales of woe. It could have encouraged me to do the right things because I would have had evidence that not everything has to go bad. Wellness could have been documented— not just hoped for. Good news can provide a justification for optimism. Some sense of wellness can provide a realistic basis for striving for further wellness. A sense of success can breed more success. It becomes a happy continuum: good news leads to a good attitude which leads to a positive approach which results in better health which is good news.

What had happened to me? Why was I so susceptible to despair? What had prevented me from enjoying earlier the benefits of my good news? Why did I have to rely upon a friend who had the insight and the motivation to seek out and to relay the good news?

First, I probably did not ask about the medical tests that I had not heard about. Apparently, I had assumed the "half-empty" perspective. I probably focused upon the bad news—the things that the hospital personnel were anxious to find and to treat. I may have purposely ignored the missing information—not wishing to ask about something else that might be wrong. I may not have heard the good news when it was told to me. My apprehensions, if not terror, of complications could have totally overshadowed any good news that was told to me. My pessimism might not have allowed any nurturing of hope.

Second, those around me—whether my family or the health-care professionals—may not have ensured that I had heard the good news. They may not have told me. Hospitals and doctors' offices can be hectic places with so many patients and so many duties that there might not have been the opportunity to relay the details of "normal" test results. Also doctors and nurses tend to focus upon problems. They want to help solve medical problems by identifying the problem, suggesting the solution, and helping to implement the treatment procedure. Good news, thus, is not in the forefront of their consciousness. Plus they may be too accustomed to dealing with "half-empty" (or worse) situations with patients. People in hospitals or doctors' offices have a tendency to be ill; wellness frequently isn't a major topic of conversation. Also, sometimes the health-care professionals do not notice that the good news isn't sinking in for the patient. Patients tend to nod, smile, agree, and say that they understand what they are being told under any condition. Add a mixture of good news and bad news, and it is no mystery which news will be remembered.

Having a disease is nothing to celebrate. However, to succumb to a pessimistic, "half-empty" attitude toward the disease and therefore to life does not make sense. At the very least, it can obstruct the effective handling of the disease. At the very worst, it can poison the entire life of the person with the disease. On the other hand, a "half-full," optimistic attitude can contribute to the successful treatment of the disease and initiate a cycle of accomplishment. A positive approach can create an optimism which can nurture wellness in one's life as well in the treatment of the disease.

Treating those with diabetes also can be disheartening. It is almost as important that the health-care professionals remain positive and optimistic. Their attitude influences their patients' approach: their positive attitude will help patients work for wellness.

It also can make the job easier by helping the doctors, nurses, and nutritionists see what they succeed at rather than focusing upon their disappointments.

It just makes sense to look for the good news, to believe in the good news, and to spread the good news.

So, what's the good news?

Only Yourself

Recently a doctor and a nurse got involved in a heated discussion about responsibility for the therapeutic alliance in diabetes care.

One side of the discussion suggested that it is the health-care professional who bears primary responsibility for getting the alliance to work. The nurse felt that the doctor, the nurse, the counselor, or the nutritionist must search continually for the "right button" to push. Through undaunted persistence or altering strategies or some other ingredient, one of the medical members of the health-care team continually seeks to fulfill his other obligations to the patient and to the Hippocratic Oath. The implication of this position was that the obligation never ends.

The other side of the discussion declined to assume primary responsibility for the effectiveness of the diabetes treatment. While not resorting to the actual worn phrases, the doctor suggested essentially that "you can take a horse to water but you can't make it drink" and that "one can only do so much." As well as citing the medical profession's limitations of time and energy, he questioned the value of assuming the burden of—or any portion thereof—someone else's disease. The implication of this position was that the patient—not the health-care professional—must assume the obligation for the diabetes.

The doctor and the nurse parted without resolving their disagreement.

I believe that a person with diabetes must depend only on himself or herself. Therefore, in my opinion, the responsibility for diabetes rests with the person with the disease. It is his or her obligation.

My opinion extends well beyond professional health care. The person with diabetes must depend only on himself or herself. He/she must see the rest of the professional and non-professional health-care team at best as *trying* to help.

Perhaps my position sounds harsh, cold, arrogant, and ungrateful. Nevertheless, I feel that the person with the disease has the most reliable source about his/her disease—himself/herself—and therefore must act primarily on the basis of that source.

Consider the other members of the health-care team who might assume the obligation or the responsibility for the therapeutic program. The medical community of doctors, nurses, nutritionists, and others know more about medicine in general and diabetes in particular. But their knowledge is of the *usual* or *typical* patient. They know what happens most frequently and what most often is done to treat the disease. They are dealing with the statistical average—the rule rather than the exception. Surely that is the best way when you are treating a number of patients.

But it is the patient who knows what he/she feels, what the symptoms are, and how severe they are. He/she must provide the data which will, in turn, determine whether his/her case fits the rule or is the exception. He/she must be responsible for providing the data. It must be accurate, objective, and immediate. He/she should not relinquish this obligation in hopes that the doctor or the nurse will assume it. This is no easy task. People worry about making others angry, about being a crybaby, about what the treatment might cost, and about what it all means. But, in reality, without objective data, the medical profession is essentially guessing. The patient has to depend upon himself/herself to provide the facts if the diagnosis, the treatment, and the prognosis are to be correct.

The remainder of the health-care team—family, friends, colleagues, counselors, and others—function in even more subjective roles. Usually without the in-depth knowledge of the disease and the extensive experience with a variety of people with diabetes, they participate in the therapeutic alliance as their particular person carries out his life. They see him/her working and playing, loving and hating, laughing and crying, succeeding and failing, eating and sleeping, coming and going. Usually none of these activities has anything to do with diabetes; sometimes they have a lot to do with the disease. Who knows? Only the person with the diabetes. Again, all the others at best are guessing.

The person with the diabetes has the best opportunity to know if his/her anger or depression is due to low sugar or to widespread incompetence at work. He/she should be the one to determine if he/she ought to climb a mountain or to have a drink. It is his/her responsibility to adjust his/her insulin, diet, or exercise. Certainly, others care—perhaps too much—but even the greatest amount of experience with a person who has diabetes is still second-hand. Even if this member of the health-care team has diabetes also, his/her diabetes is unique and thus he/she can be only so helpful. As with the medical members of the team, the non-medical members can only guess as to what is going on. The person with the diabetes has the best vantage point and therefore the best chance of knowing what is happening.

I appreciate the entire health-care team's efforts. I appreciate their knowledge, their experience, their dedication, their sincerity, their love, and their pain. I know that many would like to assume some of the burden of the disease. I appreciate that they all are trying their best and that they care.

But I am the only person who will always be there with my diabetes. I always will be able to reach myself when a decision has to be made about dosage, diet, or exercise. I can count only on myself being there when a glucose test, an injection, or a ketone test has to be done. If a crisis develops, perhaps I will be alone with my insulin reaction or will have no phone available to call my doctor and ask his advice about my fruity breath. A member of the health-care team may not always be there. People move, go on vacation, and change jobs. I have to take responsibility for the treatment of my diabetes.

I can be sure only of what is going on in my head and heart. If I am to know what motives, feelings, and environmental factors are influencing the therapeutic alliance, they can be only mine. I have no way of knowing with certainty what is making a doctor, a nurse, a wife, a son, or a friend tick at a particular time when they give advice or offer an opinion. I can only guess with some certainty what is motivating me or what is driving me or what is frightening me. To feel relatively safe, I must trust myself.

I don't know whether the doctor or the nurse is more correct about on whom the primary responsibility of the therapeutic alliance rests. For me, however, I know that I must assume the responsibility. I must learn more about the disease. I must develop a more objective way to report my symptoms. I must have more courage when dealing with the other members of the health-care team. I need to know when and where to seek help. I must assume all of the tasks involved in treating the disease daily. I must trust my feelings and judgment about my diabetes care.

It is *my* disease. I have to take responsibility for my life. I must do this because I believe that, ultimately, I must depend only on myself.

It Ain't Easy

I BEGAN WRITING *The Human Side of Diabetes* in 1983. Now, in 1991, it is time to complete this personal history of my efforts to come to terms with diabetes. Clearly, my struggle with the disease is not over. Thank goodness. But, it is time to move on to a new dimension of my life. I am trying to bring my truce with the disease and my enhanced sense of self to writing short stories about men and women, fathers and sons.

I hope that *The Human Side of Diabetes* will provide some direction for discovering a richer life for yourself. However, I will be satisfied if this book serves as a permission slip for all of us "with diabetes" to be more human. To me, being "diabetic" just isn't enough.

Much like a non-believer who recently has been converted to a faith, I tend to be zealous (overzealous?) in my urging of others to join the human side of diabetes. Like a parent anxious to spare his children from making the "mistakes" he did, I can slip easily into a string of "do" and "don't" commands. Like a person who has endured the consequences of something he wished he hadn't done, I find myself imploring others to "do as I say, not as I do."

Of course, much of what the new convert urges, the old parent commands, or the experienced person implores can sound like the cliches and platitudes we are subjected to while wrestling with a chronic disease. But *The Human Side of Diabetes* was not written as a collection of sermons, commands, or warnings. It is meant for the context of actual human experience. It insists upon the human context. If removed from that context, what this book urges, commands, and implores could sound pat, automatic, reductive, or superficial ("Just do such-and-such. . . ."); insensitive, impersonal, disconnected, or insincere ("Most people with diabetes. . . ."); or wrong-headed and unexamined ("Merely change. . . .").

I urge you not to reduce this book, the living with diabetes, or the human side of diabetes to a series of axioms to post on the refrigerator and memorize. To do so would be the same as treating your diabetes without considering who you are, what you do, and how you wish to live.

By now, you should know how I feel about that!

We are people with diabetes, not "diabetics." As people, I believe, we will be better off if we allow ourselves to experience the whole range of our emotions. We need to come out of the closet. We not only can admit to feelings such as despair, anger, disillusionment, terror, and apathy, but also should permit ourselves to express them. By sharing or communicating the "dark side," we help others know what we are going through and what is driving us. There is little to be gained by eating our emotions, by pretending that everything is "fine," or by disguising our pain. We also will help ourselves by bringing out into the open how we feel and why we feel that way. Furthermore, it seems important to celebrate the "upside": hope, victories, good news, and good feelings. Recognizing the joys in life helps us appreciate the value of living and the quality of life. Recalling the upside can help us get through the dark times. Life, we need to remind ourselves, is much more than something to get through.

As people, we are a part of a species. We are members of several communities. Not only are we among millions of people with diabetes, but we also are among the millions of those who live, work, and play in America. We are Americans, workers, children, parents, friends, co-workers, playmates, and neighbors.

While it may require some teaching about the disease, many of these people will work with us and our diabetes. They are family, friends, colleagues, and health-care providers. We can captain a team which offers a dynamic therapeutic alliance for managing the disease. Help is available for choosing ways to administer and adjust insulin, selecting a diet, developing an exercise regimen, combating complications, handling the emotional terrains, and using a wellness approach to living. We should not hesitate to utilize that help.

We should strive to be realistic in the handling of the chronic disease. By understanding the vagaries of diabetes, accepting what we have learned, and accommodating ourselves as best as possible to those vagaries, we can enhance the quality of our lives. But be careful not to expect too much. Rarely is a journey without bumps, bruises, and detours. Progress on the road toward a richer life frequently is slow going and requires perpetual adjustment and adaptation. We are human, and humans aren't perfect. No health-care team or therapeutic alliance made up of humans will be perfect or do perfect work. It makes no sense to be harsh with anyone on the team or with any genuine effort by team members, including ourselves. Try to relax, but certainly be gentle.

Rather than being controlled by the disease or letting the issue of control dominate us, we should assume control of our lives. While a therapeutic alliance with a health-care team can offer external resources, we need to cultivate and to depend upon our internal resources. Diabetes is nothing to be ashamed of. We should emerge from the closet and live. Once out of that "diabetic" closet, we owe it to ourselves to live actively. Having diabetes does not mean that we have to be passive. Choices are to be made. By examining the alternatives, weighing our options, and making informed decisions, we empower ourselves. Each decision we make establishes that it is our life and that we have control of it. The opportunities are limitless: we can choose the members of our health-care team, the form of glucose monitoring, the type of diet, the variety of exercise, the method for glucose control, the attitude toward life and diabetes, and the ways for coping. The process of making choices and taking responsibility for those choices ensures that we are living our own lives.

We can all benefit by working to live today and to look to the future. Because the treatment of diabetes seems preoccupied with the past—what did you eat, how much insulin or medication did you take, how long did you exercise, what was your last blood glucose, how long have you had diabetes?—and because many seem to focus on the limitations associated with the disease, this paradoxical focus on today and tomorrow, perhaps, seems difficult. I don't think so. First, the past is gone. It's done. There's nothing we can do about yesterday's HA1C, ice cream, or doctor's appointment. Second, we are not condemned to repeat the past. As humans we can learn and change. We can read, ask advice, and pay attention to our experiences. Rather than punishing ourselves over what has happened, we can use the past to live better now. Third, the promise of a future is a substantial reward. Living well now not only has its immediate benefits, but also offers hope for a tomorrow and for living well tomorrow. Hope in general and hope for a future seem ample motivation for doing what needs to be done as we live with diabetes. The sooner we start having an investment in the future the greater the opportunity for dividends for realizing that hope.

However, as we all know, there are no guarantees. That's what makes living and living with diabetes so difficult.

It takes work. A tremendous effort is required to come out of the closet, to become an active leader of a therapeutic alliance, to maintain realistic expectations, to take responsibility for your life, and to have faith in a future.

It takes dedication. Diabetes is a 24-hour-a-day disease. There are no vacations. Very little in life doesn't affect it. We always are either doing something connected to managing diabetes or thinking about what we might be doing.

It takes courage. Despite all the work and all the sincerity in the world, there are no assurances. Even if we were to do "all the right things"—what are they? who could do them all right?—we cannot count on wellness or even tomorrow. One has to be brave to do the work without some certainty of justice and/or mercy.

In a phrase, it ain't easy.

Living with diabetes ain't easy.

Maintaining the human side of diabetes ain't easy.

But I urge you to live with your diabetes and to stake your claim on the human side of the disease.

After these last eight years, I am convinced more than ever that there are more and more ways to come to terms with a chronic disease like diabetes. This book has ventured what I have come up with, what I have learned from others, and what I have tried for 36 years.

Now I challenge you to try out my strategies for joining the human side of diabetes. I challenge you to develop your own strategies. I challenge you share your experiences with others. I urge you to become a living permission slip for others—whether they have diabetes or not—to venture to the human side of diabetes and to nurture the human side of living.

I am convinced that it can make all the difference. It has for me.

Index

About the Author

Born in Flushing, New York, Michael Raymond learned his American geography as his parents "relocated" seventeen times before he finished high school. He developed insulin-dependent diabetes at age nine in 1955 and has experienced a wide array of health-care experiences since his first visit to the Elliot P. Joslin Clinic in Boston. Married with two sons, he is a professor of English at Stetson University in DeLand, Florida. Having earned an M.A. in black American fiction and a Ph.D. in eighteenth-century British fiction at the University of Florida, he prefers teaching modern fiction, writing, and freshman English. His 19 years at Stetson have included "careers" and publications in business communications, the educational application of computers in language arts and patient education, teacher training, creative writing, and diabetes care. A founding member of STS (the Stetson Teleological Society), Mike enjoys poker, sports, and watching the "taillights of his sons Eric and Bryan as they become more and more successful writers, musicians, and humans." He looks to a future of "immediate fame and fortune" as a fictionist and of being a grandfather in about 15 years.